2nd Edition

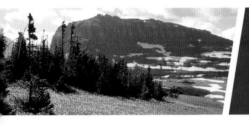

BEST ⛺ **TENT**
Camping

MONTANA

YOUR CAR-CAMPING GUIDE TO SCENIC BEAUTY, THE SOUNDS
OF NATURE, AND AN ESCAPE FROM CIVILIZATION

To Silva and Aleksia, our beloved daughters, whose love, precious spirits, and inspiration make every journey fun and memorable.

—Jan and Christina Nesset

Best Tent Camping: Montana
Copyright © 2017 by Jan and Christina Nesset
All rights reserved
Printed in the United States of America
Published by Menasha Ridge Press
Distributed by Publishers Group West
Second edition, first printing

Library of Congress Cataloging-in-Publication Data

Names: Soderberg, Vicky, author. | Soderberg, Ken, author. | Nesset, Jan, author. | Nesset, Christina, author.
Title: Best tent camping : Montana / Ken and Vicky Soderberg ; updated by Jan and Christina Nesset.
Description: Second edition. | Birmingham, Alabama : Menasha Ridge Press, [2017] | First edition: 2005. |
     "Distributed by Publishers Group West"—T.p. verso.
Identifiers: LCCN 2016057900 | ISBN 978-1-63404-002-0 (paperback) | ISBN 978-1-63404-003-7 (e-book)
Subjects: LCSH: Camping—Montana—Guidebooks. | Camp sites, facilities, etc.—Montana—Guidebooks. |
     Outdoor recreation. | Montana—Guidebooks.
Classification: LCC GV191.42.M9 S63 2017 | DDC 917.86/068—dc23
LC record available at lccn.loc.gov/2016057900

Project editor: Ritchey Halphen
Cover design: Scott McGrew
Maps: Steve Jones, Jan and Christina Nesset
Book design: Jonathan Norberg
Photos: Jan and Christina Nesset, except where noted
Editors: Susan Roberts McWilliams *(copy)*, Dan Downing *(research)*
Proofreader: Scott Alexander Jones
Indexer: Sylvia Coates

MENASHA RIDGE PRESS
An imprint of AdventureKEEN
2204 First Ave. S., Ste. 102
Birmingham, Alabama 35233
800-443-7227, fax 205-326-1012

Visit menasharidge.com for a complete listing of our books and for ordering information. Contact us at our website, at facebook.com/menasharidge, or at twitter.com/menasharidge with questions or comments. To find out more about who we are and what we're doing, visit blog.menasharidge.com.

Front cover: Reynolds Creek and Reynolds Mountain in Glacier National Park are located near the Going-to-the-Sun Road, which takes you to Sprague Creek Campground (page 45). *Photo:* Kerrick James/Alamy Stock Photo

2nd Edition

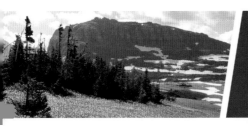

BEST TENT Camping

MONTANA

YOUR CAR-CAMPING GUIDE TO SCENIC BEAUTY, THE SOUNDS
OF NATURE, AND AN ESCAPE FROM CIVILIZATION

Jan and Christina Nesset

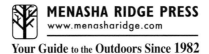

MENASHA RIDGE PRESS
www.menasharidge.com

Your Guide to the Outdoors Since 1982

Montana Campground Locator Map

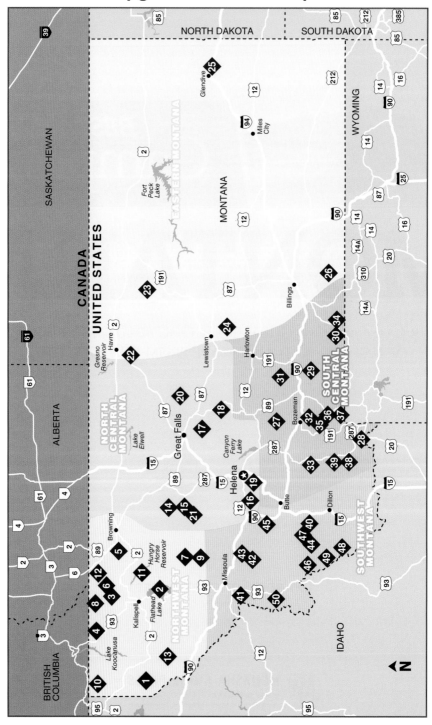

CONTENTS

Montana Campground Locator Map . . . . opposite page

Map Legend vii

Acknowledgments viii

Preface ix

Best Campgrounds x

Introduction 1

NORTHWEST MONTANA 11

1 Bad Medicine Campground 12

2 Big Arm Unit–Flathead Lake State Park Campground 15

3 Big Creek Campground 18

4 Big Therriault Lake Campground 21

5 Cut Bank Campground 24

6 Fish Creek Campground 27

7 Holland Lake Campground 30

8 Kintla Lake Campground 33

9 Lake Alva Campground 36

10 Pete Creek Campground 39

11 Peters Creek Campground 42

12 Sprague Creek Campground 45

13 Thompson Falls State Park Campground 48

NORTH CENTRAL MONTANA 51

14 Cave Mountain Campground 52

15 Home Gulch Campground 55

16 Kading Campground 58

17 Logging Creek Campground 61

18 Many Pines Campground 64

19 Park Lake Campground 67

20 Thain Creek Campground 70

21 Wood Lake Campground 73

EASTERN MONTANA 76

22 Beaver Creek County Park Campgrounds. 77

23 Camp Creek Campground 80

24 Crystal Lake Campground 83

25 Makoshika State Park Campground 86

26 Sage Creek Campground. 91

SOUTH CENTRAL MONTANA 93

27 Battle Ridge Campground 94

28 Beaver Creek Campground. 97

29 Falls Creek Campground 100

30 Greenough Lake Campground 103

31 Halfmoon Campground. 106

32 Hood Creek Campground. 109

33 Potosi Campground. 112

34 Sheridan Campground 115

35 Spire Rock Campground 118

36 Swan Creek Campground 121

37 Tom Miner Campground 124

38 Wade and Cliff Lakes Area Campgrounds 127

39 West Fork Madison Dispersed Sites 130

SOUTHWEST MONTANA 133

40 Bannack State Park Campground. 134

41 Charles Waters Campground 137

42 Dalles Campground 140

43 Grasshopper Campground 143

44 Lost Creek State Park Campground 146

45 Martin Creek Campground 149

46 May Creek Campground 152

47 Miner Lake Campground 155

48 Reservoir Lake Campground 158

49 Twin Lakes Campground 161

50 Three Frogs Campground. 164

APPENDIX A: Camping-Equipment Checklist 167

APPENDIX B: Sources of Information 168

Index 170

About the Authors 177

Map Legend

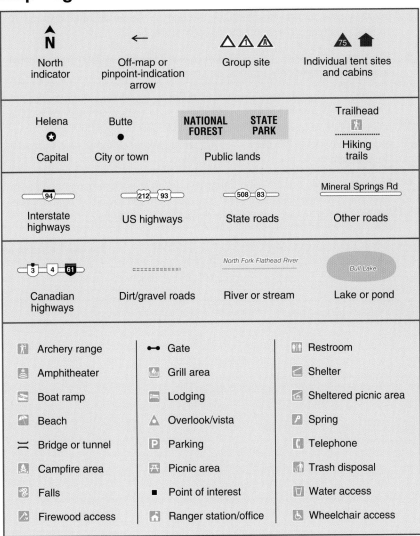

ACKNOWLEDGMENTS

The authors wish to thank the following people:

- The busy, hardworking state and federal employees who volunteered their precious time to provide feedback, dredge up resources, and respond to countless inquiries to support the revision of this book.

- The Covington family, who enthusiastically took on "assignments" to visit campgrounds, take photographs, and review information.

- The crews of the Montana Conservation Corps, who toiled in the mountains to reduce forest fuel hazards, restore and build trails, and enhance wildlife habitat while graciously fact-checking details and maps at and near campgrounds featured in this book, many of which were their temporary homes for the summer.

- Silva and Aleksia, our amazing daughters, for their encouragement, support, love, and patience while Mom and Dad steered them toward visits to on-the-way and out-of-the-way campgrounds and fun spots nearby.

—Jan and Christina Nesset

PREFACE

This book is simply a new layer put to the excellent work of the original authors, Ken and Vicky Soderberg, who traveled all over Montana for the singular purpose of seeking the state's best tent camping. In digging into the material for this revision, and after spinning off some miles to explore the first of many campgrounds, we quickly learned that the original book was more than a spilling of the beans—it was a labor of love. Our hats are off to the Soderbergs for turning us on to some terrific campgrounds, many previously unknown to us!

We went about revising the book in a far different way: we built upon our years of tent camping across this amazing state by exploring new-to-us territory, with the hope of verifying or updating original information and finding enchanted campgrounds for tenters. We did both, and we loved every minute of it!

Jan was raised in eastern Montana and moved continually westward across the state to get his education. His father was fond of fishing, which meant that most family vacations were spent near bodies of water not far from either a camper or a small trailer. The kids, however, opted frequently for a pup tent. As a young adult, Jan reveled in outdoor pursuits, in particular climbing, paddling, bicycling, and adventure racing. His itch for travel took him around the planet, with either a backpack or bicycle panniers stuffed with gear. And always a tent!

Chris spent her childhood exploring the Blue Ridge Mountains of Virginia and frolicking along the beaches of the Atlantic Ocean. Her first job out of college was in public-land conservation, which gave her the opportunity to take her outdoor interests and test them during an exploration of the West. Plus, her work and chosen lifestyle had her frequently living out of a tent.

Chris met Jan on a beach during a surfing weekend in Oregon, and they got married two years later on that same beach, after going surfing. For their honeymoon, they loaded bicycles and toured the Andes of South America for six months. They lived out of a tent the entire trip, with the exception of the occasional breaks for showers and clean clothes.

Our marriage is how this book materialized—through the collective preferences, quirks, and biases of two people who not only love getting outdoors but who also prefer camping in tents over camping by means that are towed, carried, or driven.

We hope that you find some comfort in knowing that the people who wrote this book are biased in your favor, having accumulated decades of actual experience—complete with plenty of mistakes, serendipity, dumb luck, and doses of hard-won savvy (toot!) in the field.

BEST CAMPGROUNDS

BEST FOR MOUNTAIN BIKING

14 Cave Mountain Campground **North Central Montana** (p. 52)

15 Home Gulch Campground **North Central Montana** (p. 55)

16 Kading Campground **North Central Montana** (p. 58)

17 Logging Creek Campground **North Central Montana** (p. 61)

19 Park Lake Campground **North Central Montana** (p. 67)

24 Crystal Lake Campground **Eastern Montana** (p. 83)

27 Battle Ridge Campground **South Central Montana** (p. 94)

34 Sheridan Campground **South Central Montana** (p. 115)

41 Charles Waters Campground **Southwest Montana** (p. 137)

48 Reservoir Lake Campground **Southwest Montana** (p. 158)

BEST FOR FISHING

1 Bad Medicine Campground **Northwest Montana** (p. 12)

2 Big Arm Unit–Flathead Lake State Park Campground **Northwest Montana** (p. 15)

3 Big Creek Campground **Northwest Montana** (p. 18)

7 Holland Lake Campground **Northwest Montana** (p. 30)

8 Kintla Lake Campground **Northwest Montana** (p. 33)

9 Lake Alva Campground **Northwest Montana** (p. 36)

13 Thompson Falls State Park Campground **Northwest Montana** (p. 48)

14 Cave Mountain Campground **North Central Montana** (p. 52)

15 Home Gulch Campground **North Central Montana** (p. 55)

19 Park Lake Campground **North Central Montana** (p. 67)

21 Wood Lake Campground **North Central Montana** (p. 73)

22 Beaver Creek County Park Campgrounds **Eastern Montana** (p. 77)

28 Beaver Creek Campground **South Central Montana** (p. 97)

29 Falls Creek Campground **South Central Montana** (p. 100)

30 Greenough Lake Campground **South Central Montana** (p. 103)

32 Hood Creek Campground **South Central Montana** (p. 109)

36 Swan Creek Campground **South Central Montana** (p. 121)

38 Wade and Cliff Lakes Area Campgrounds **South Central Montana** (p. 127)

42 Dalles Campground **Southwest Montana** (p. 140)

47 Miner Lake Campground **Southwest Montana** (p. 155)

48 Reservoir Lake Campground **Southwest Montana** (p. 158)

49 Twin Lakes Campground **Southwest Montana** (p. 161)

50 Three Frogs Campground **Southwest Montana** (p. 164)

BEST FOR FAMILIES WITH KIDS

2   Big Arm Unit–Flathead Lake State Park Campground **Northwest Montana** (p. 15)

6   Fish Creek Campground **Northwest Montana** (p. 27)

7   Holland Lake Campground **Northwest Montana** (p. 30)

13 Thompson Falls State Park Campground **Northwest Montana** (p. 48)

16 Kading Campground **North Central Montana** (p. 58)

17 Logging Creek Campground **North Central Montana** (p. 61)

19 Park Lake Campground **North Central Montana** (p. 67)

22 Beaver Creek County Park Campgrounds **Eastern Montana** (p. 77)

30 Greenough Lake Campground **South Central Montana** (p. 103)

38 Wade and Cliff Lakes Area Campgrounds **South Central Montana** (p. 127)

40 Bannack State Park Campground **Southwest Montana** (p. 134)

48 Reservoir Lake Campground **Southwest Montana** (p. 158)

50 Three Frogs Campground **Southwest Montana** (p. 164)

BEST FOR HIKING

1   Bad Medicine Campground **Northwest Montana** (p. 12)

11 Peters Creek Campground **Northwest Montana** (p. 42)

14 Cave Mountain Campground **North Central Montana** (p. 52)

15 Home Gulch Campground **North Central Montana** (p. 55)

16 Kading Campground **North Central Montana** (p. 58)

20 Thain Creek Campground **North Central Montana** (p. 70)

21 Wood Lake Campground **North Central Montana** (p. 73)

24 Crystal Lake Campground **Eastern Montana** (p. 83)

27 Battle Ridge Campground **South Central Montana** (p. 94)

31 Halfmoon Campground **South Central Montana** (p. 106)

32 Hood Creek Campground **South Central Montana** (p. 109)

33 Potosi Campground **South Central Montana** (p. 112)

35 Spire Rock Campground **South Central Montana** (p. 118)

41 Charles Waters Campground **Southwest Montana** (p. 137)

43 Grasshopper Campground **Southwest Montana** (p. 143)

46 May Creek Campground **Southwest Montana** (p. 152)

47 Miner Lake Campground **Southwest Montana** (p. 155)

48 Reservoir Lake Campground **Southwest Montana** (p. 158)

50 Three Frogs Campground **Southwest Montana** (p. 164)

BEST FOR PADDLING

8 Kintla Lake Campground **Northwest Montana** (p. 33)

9 Lake Alva Campground **Northwest Montana** (p. 36)

13 Thompson Falls State Park Campground **Northwest Montana** (p. 48)

19 Park Lake Campground **North Central Montana** (p. 67)

21 Wood Lake Campground **North Central Montana** (p. 73)

23 Camp Creek Campground **Eastern Montana** (p. 80)

24 Crystal Lake Campground **Eastern Montana** (p. 83)

32 Hood Creek Campground **South Central Montana** (p. 109)

38 Wade and Cliff Lakes Area Campgrounds **South Central Montana** (p. 127)

47 Miner Lake Campground **Southwest Montana** (p. 155)

48 Reservoir Lake Campground **Southwest Montana** (p. 158)

49 Twin Lakes Campground **Southwest Montana** (p. 161)

BEST FOR PRIVACY AND SOLITUDE

4 Big Therriault Lake Campground **Northwest Montana** (p. 21)

26 Sage Creek Campground **Eastern Montana** (p. 91)

33 Potosi Campground **South Central Montana** (p. 112)

35 Spire Rock Campground **South Central Montana** (p. 118)

43 Grasshopper Campground **Southwest Montana** (p. 143)

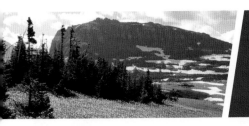

2nd Edition

BEST **TENT**
Camping

MONTANA

YOUR CAR-CAMPING GUIDE TO SCENIC BEAUTY, THE SOUNDS
OF NATURE, AND AN ESCAPE FROM CIVILIZATION

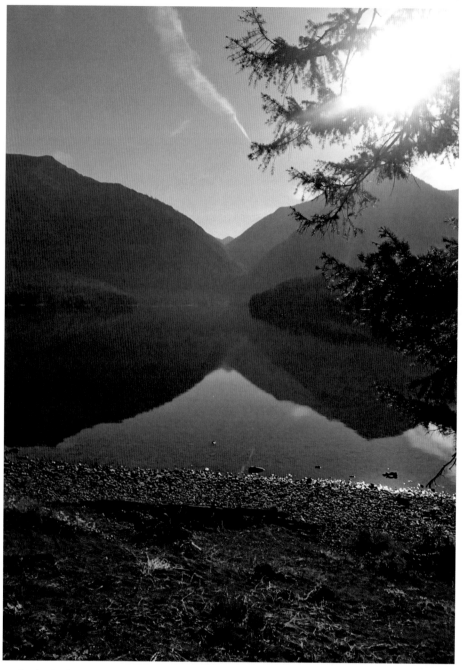

Holland Lake *(see Holland Lake Campground, page 30)*

INTRODUCTION

HOW TO USE THIS GUIDEBOOK

Menasha Ridge Press welcomes you to *Best Tent Camping: Montana*. Whether you're new to camping or you've been sleeping in your portable shelter over decades of outdoor adventures, please review the following information. It explains how we have worked with the author to organize this book and how you can make the best use of it.

Some passages in this introduction are applicable to all of the books in the Best Tent Camping series. Where this isn't the case, such as in the descriptions of weather, wildlife, and plants, the authors have provided information specific to the area covered in this particular book.

THE RATING SYSTEM

As with all books in the Best Tent Camping series, this guidebook's authors personally experienced dozens of campgrounds and campsites to select the top 50 locations in this region. Within that universe of 50 sites, the authors then ranked each one according to the six categories described below.

Each campground is superlative in its own way. For example, a site may be rated only one star in one category but perhaps five stars in another category. Our rating system allows you to choose your destination based on the attributes that are most important to you. Although these ratings are subjective, they're still excellent guidelines for finding the perfect camping experience for you and your companions.

Below and following, we describe the criteria for each of the attributes in our five-star rating system:

★★★★★ The site is **ideal** in that category.

★★★★ The site is **exemplary** in that category.

★★★ The site is **very good** in that category.

★★ The site is **above average** in that category.

INDIVIDUAL RATINGS

Each of the campground descriptions includes ratings for **beauty, site privacy, site spaciousness, quiet, security,** and **cleanliness**; each attribute is ranked from one to five stars, with five being the best. Yes, these ratings are subjective, but we've tried to select campgrounds that offer something for everyone.

Beauty

Exceptional scenery is practically a given throughout Montana, but five-star sites will provide excellent views, and you will know you're in a special place. The campground will be oriented to blend with and complement its natural surroundings, with the sounds and smells of nature rounding out the experience.

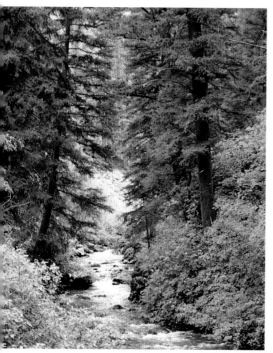
Storm Castle Creek, near Spire Rock Campground
(see page 118)

Site Privacy

Ideally, any trees, shrubs, and boulders or other natural features will be left in place or incorporated into the site development to offer privacy and barriers between adjacent sites. The best campgrounds have well-spaced sites, with little visual contact between neighbors and a sense of solitude due to the campground's distance from the nearest roads and towns.

Quiet

Our top rating for quiet means you'll find little or no overhead or road noise, minimal social noise, an aura of solitude, and quiet hours enforced by staff (if there is any staff). It was a plus if we could hear the water from a nearby river or stream, the songs of birds, or the wind through the trees. Admittedly, quiet is a difficult attribute to quantify because it can change quickly depending on your neighbor.

Site Spaciousness

Spacious to us means plenty of room for two tents to be set back from the parking area and away from the fire ring. There should also be space for separate areas to cook, eat, and just kick back without being on top of your neighbors.

Security

Many sites have no on-site host, but those that do and those where there is cell phone coverage received higher ratings. We also checked for an absence of vandalism.

Cleanliness

Everyone wants to see restrooms, fire pits, and picnic tables that are clean and a campground free of ground litter. If the site was well maintained—signs were in good repair and were up to date, buildings were in good repair, and roads were maintained—then the campground received high marks. Signs of noxious weeds that were out of control resulted in a lower rating.

THE CAMPGROUND PROFILE

Each profile contains a concise but informative narrative that describes the campground and individual sites. Readers get a sense not only of the property itself but also the recreational opportunities available nearby. This descriptive text is enhanced with three helpful sidebars: Ratings, Key Information, and Getting There (accurate driving directions that lead you to the campground from the nearest major roadway).

THE CAMPGROUND LOCATOR MAP AND MAP LEGEND

Use the Montana Campground Locator Map, on page iv, to assess the exact location of each campground. The campground's number appears not only on the overview map but also in the table of contents, and on the profile's first page.

A map legend that details the symbols found on the campground-layout maps appears on page vii.

CAMPGROUND-LAYOUT MAPS

Each profile includes a detailed map of campground sites, internal roads, facilities, and other key items.

GPS CAMPGROUND-ENTRANCE COORDINATES

Readers can easily access all campgrounds in this book by using the directions given and the overview map, which shows at least one major road leading into the area. But for those who enjoy using GPS technology to navigate, the book includes coordinates for each campground's entrance in latitude and longitude, expressed in degrees and decimal minutes.

To convert GPS coordinates from degrees, minutes, and seconds to the above degree–decimal minute format, the seconds are divided by 60. For more on GPS technology, visit usgs.gov.

A note of caution: Actual GPS devices will easily guide you to any of these campgrounds, but users of smartphone mapping apps may find that cell phone service is often unavailable in the remote areas where many of these hideaways are located.

ABOUT THIS BOOK

Montana is a big state—don't be fooled by its relative size in an atlas. The reality is that 53 of its 56 counties are individually bigger than Rhode Island, and it's farther from Yaak to Alzada in Montana than it is from Washington, DC, to Chicago or to Jacksonville, Florida. On top of that, this immense state has more elbow room than you might expect, having hit a population of one million people only in 2011. (It's neck and neck, but as of this writing, even Rhode Island has more people.)

With all this room to roam, travel in Montana is an exhilarating adventure.

In exploring this immense state, we as authors have experienced flat tires, blown engines, and closed roads, as well as unexpected sightings of bighorn sheep, mountain goats, moose, and bears. We've followed roads on the highway map that were nothing more than tire ruts and awakened to six inches of snow in August, subfreezing temperatures in July, and seemingly endless days of sunshine. We can also confirm that when a tree falls in the woods, it *does* make a sound (in one case, too near a campsite).

Montana is also a landscape of breathtaking diversity. Did you know there are 64 distinct mountain ranges in Montana? We have stood atop the Continental Divide and many of this state's highest peaks, including Granite Peak, Montana's highest point at 12,807 feet above sea level. We've hiked trails in the Beartooths, the Bitterroots, the Cabinets, the Crazies, the Big Belts, the Bridgers, the Gravellys, the Tendoys, the Tobacco Roots, and the Missions, and spent time backpacking in Glacier and Yellowstone Parks and the Bob Marshall Wilderness Area. We've also paddled some of Montana's great waterways, including either placid or whitewater river stretches of the Yellowstone, Gallatin, Madison, Bitterroot, Little Blackfoot, Missouri, and Yaak Rivers, as well as forks of the Flathead River, along with too many lakes and ponds to count. Each has its own unique characteristic and the promise of something new and spectacular to witness.

We'll never tire of seeing spring wildflowers or watching waterfalls created by the icy-cold spring runoff. We welcome summer-afternoon thunderstorms that roll across the sky, drench us, and leave behind spectacular rainbows. We marvel at cool fall days with their splashes of yellows and oranges set against the deep-blue sky, and we can even appreciate those winter weekends when the temperature swings from 30 above on Friday to 30 below by Saturday afternoon.

Yes, Montana is a land of extremes. Summers are typically warm and dry, but you should be prepared for any kind of weather. Snow in July is not uncommon at higher elevations, and sudden rainstorms can make roads dangerous and impassable. The same type of hailstorms that menaced the Lewis and Clark Expedition may pummel your outing. It's nothing to worry about, though, if you are prepared and take proper precautions.

Being prepared is a constant challenge, since being totally prepared for every possibility would involve more gear than any vehicle can hold. Planning ahead and getting current information is key. Check the weather report and contact local agencies (remembering that most are only open on weekdays). State-road conditions are available 24 hours a day by calling **511** from any phone.

Cell phone coverage in Montana, while much better than it was in 2005, when the first edition of this book was published, is nonetheless spotty to nonexistent in some parts of the state. Once you get off the interstates and away from the bigger cities, prepare for the possibility of losing signal.

Finally, note that the best thing about this book is the fun you'll have exploring new places and tenting in new campgrounds—we hope this opens up to you as never before this great state and its regions. We sure had fun revising this book, and taking turns exploring and camping in this great state, in order to put our respective touches to what we hope is a resource you'll use for years to come.

Enjoy!

WEATHER

Four distinct seasons are enjoyed under Montana's big sky, and there's truth behind the humor that each season is as unreliable as the next. Montana weather is indeed predictably unpredictable, with unseasonably cold or warm conditions possible during any season.

Spring is typically the rainy time of the year in Montana, although snowfall can and does fall throughout the spring. The statewide average annual rainfall is near 20 inches and can exceed 80 inches in the higher Rockies.

Summers are typically warm and dry, with average summer highs approaching 70 degrees across the lower elevations in central and eastern Montana. Cooler conditions are typical in the higher elevations of the Mountain West.

Fall weather commonly starts in late September and runs into November. Highly variable temperature changes can occur throughout the fall, from Indian-summer temperatures in the 60s to cold and freezing temperatures accompanied by rain and snow.

Winter temperatures can drop to 50 below zero or rise to 50 degrees above zero. The average winter snowfall in Montana is nearly 40 inches, with some mountainous regions reaching substantially deeper snowpack of more than 100 inches.

FIRST AID KIT

A useful first aid kit may contain more items than you might think necessary. These are just the basics. Prepackaged kits in waterproof bags (Atwater Carey and Adventure Medical make them) are available. As a preventive measure, take along sunscreen and insect repellent. Even though quite a few items are listed here, they pack down into a small space:

- Ace bandages or Spenco joint wraps
- Adhesive bandages, such as Band-Aids
- Antibiotic ointment (Neosporin or the generic equivalent)
- Antiseptic or disinfectant, such as Betadine or hydrogen peroxide
- Aspirin, acetaminophen (Tylenol), or ibuprofen (Advil)
- Benadryl or the generic equivalent, diphenhydramine (in case of allergic reactions)
- Butterfly-closure bandages
- Comb and tweezers (for removing ticks from your skin)
- Epinephrine in a prefilled syringe (for severe allergic reactions to outdoor mishaps such as bee stings)
- Gauze (one roll and six 4-by-4-inch compress pads)
- LED flashlight or headlamp
- Matches or lighter

- Moist towelettes
- Moleskin/Spenco 2nd Skin
- Pocketknife or multipurpose tool
- Waterproof first aid tape
- Whistle (it's more effective at signaling rescuers than your voice)

ANIMAL AND PLANT HAZARDS

Mother Nature has plenty of room to spread her wings and roots across the fourth largest state in the country. The state's vast variety of habitats attracts a great diversity of plants and animals. And visitors, too. You will spend most if not all of your time enjoying the diversity, but be aware. Several notable species of animals, along with one plant, can pose hazards.

BEARS

Bears are found on the slopes and in the canyons and valleys of the mountainous forest regions of Montana. They've even been seen on the prairies along the Rocky Mountain Front. You'll be lucky, however, to see one outside of Yellowstone National Park, but don't count on it.

Montana is home to both grizzlies and black bears. Both species will avoid humans unless food or their cubs are involved, or they're startled.

Take precautions in bear country by keeping your campsite clean and clear of food temptations, carrying pepper spray and knowing how to use it on the trail, and moving through bear country in groups and not in silence. If you do encounter a bear, remain calm and ready to use your bear spray. Make yourself look larger by raising your pack above your head and by sticking with your group. There is a lot to know about safe practices and behavior in bear country, so educate yourself before entering it.

WOLVES

Wolves are wary and have a natural fear of humans. Attacks by wolves are extremely rare, but they have happened. On the off chance that you do encounter a wolf that poses a threat, stay calm and don't run. As with bears, make yourself look larger and tighten your group. If the wolf holds a threatening stance, back away slowly and maintain eye contact.

MOUNTAIN LIONS

Stealthy and shy, the mountain lion is another predator you will be lucky to see. If you do find yourself within striking distance of a mountain lion that does not immediately retreat, stand your ground. As with bears and wolves, look large and stick together. Don't run—that makes the mountain lion's natural hunting instincts kick in. If the cat attacks, *fight*.

RATTLESNAKES

The Western rattlesnake, also known as the prairie rattler, is Montana's only venomous snake. The shy pit viper is found in open, arid country but is also fond of ponderosa pine stands and mixed grass and forest habitats. It looks for rock outcrops on south-facing slopes to den. The rule of thumb is to avoid these snakes: they're docile creatures not at all looking to bother you, so don't bother them. If you encounter one, give it a wide berth.

TICKS

Ticks are found in wooded areas throughout Montana, especially from spring to midsummer. You can contract Rocky Mountain spotted fever, Colorado tick fever, tularemia, and tick-borne relapsing fever from these annoying little critters, but it rarely happens, especially if you're vigilant and remove them soon after they find you.

Wearing light-colored clothing makes ticks easier to spot, and an insect repellent with DEET helps keep them away. Ticks crawl up shrubs and grasses and wait for people or animals to come near where their outstretched legs can grab on. Tweezers are ideal for removing ticks that have already attached—just grab as close to the skin surface as possible, and firmly pull loose without crushing. Expect a bit of redness and itching for a few days around the bite site.

POISON IVY

Poison ivy is native to Montana and grows in rocky areas, near water, and in the foothills of the lower mountains. Brushing up against the leaves of the plant is all you need to do for the rash-causing chemical, urushiol, to cause a reaction on your skin. Within minutes of contact, the urushiol penetrates the skin, causing blisters, lesions, or red, scaly rashes. While the reactions can be different from person to person, applying a topical cortisone cream will take care of most outbreaks. In areas where poison ivy is known to or may grow, wear long pants and sleeves and keep your eyes peeled for shiny green leaves that grow in threes.

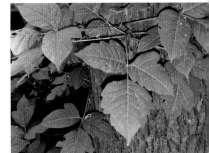

photo: *Tom Watson*

CAMPING TIPS

Car camping is a great way to see Montana. It offers the flexibility to stay places where others may not tread without forcing you to strap on a backpack. As you explore, please use camping techniques that will minimize your impact on the sites you use. Like the efforts of a careful backcountry camper, using these techniques will leave the site in good condition for the next person to enjoy.

Here are a few things to consider as you prepare for your trip:

- **PLAN AHEAD.** Know your equipment, your ability, and the area where you are camping—and prepare accordingly. Be self-sufficient at all times; carry the necessary supplies for changes in weather or other conditions. A well-executed trip is satisfying.

- **USE CARE WHEN TRAVELING.** Stay on designated roadways. Be respectful of private property and travel restrictions. Familiarize yourself with the area you'll be traveling in by picking up a map that shows land ownership. Such maps are typically available from U.S. Forest Service offices for a small fee.

- **RESERVE YOUR SITE IN ADVANCE,** especially if it's a weekend or a holiday, or if the campground is wildly popular. Many prime campgrounds require at least a six-month lead time on reservations. Check before you go.

  When selecting a site, consider your space requirements and match the site to your needs. Try to keep your group size small. If you're traveling in a large group, consider splitting up so that no more than eight people are at a single campsite. Wear and tear on a site with a large group of people can be significant even if you stay only a short time.

- **CHECK IN, PAY YOUR FEE, AND MARK YOUR SITE AS DIRECTED.** Don't just grab a seemingly empty site that looks more appealing than yours—it could be reserved. If you're unhappy with the site you've selected, check with the campground host for other options.

- **PICK YOUR CAMPING BUDDIES WISELY.** A family trip is pretty straight-forward, but you may want to reconsider including grumpy Uncle Fred, who doesn't like bugs, sunshine, or marshmallows. After you know who's going, make sure that everyone is on the same page regarding expectations of dif-ficulty (amenities or the lack thereof, physical exertion, and so on), sleeping arrangements, and food requirements.

- **DRESS FOR THE SEASON.** Educate yourself on the temperature highs and lows of the specific part of the state you plan to visit. It may be warm at night in the summer in your backyard, but up in the mountains it will be quite chilly.

- **PITCH YOUR TENT ON A LEVEL SURFACE,** preferably one covered with leaves, pine straw, or grass. Use a tarp or specially designed footprint to thwart ground moisture and to protect the tent floor. Do a little site mainte-nance, such as picking up the small rocks and sticks that can damage your tent floor and make sleeping uncomfortable. If you have a separate tent rainfly but don't think you'll need it, keep it rolled up at the base of the tent in case it starts raining at midnight.

- **CONSIDER TAKING A SLEEPING PAD IF THE GROUND MAKES YOU UNCOMFORTABLE.** Choose a pad that is full length and thicker than you think you might need. This will not only keep your hips from aching on hard ground, but it will also help keep you warm. A wide range of thin, light, or inflatable pads is available at camping stores today, and these are a much bet-ter choice than home air mattresses, which conduct heat away from the body and tend to deflate during the night.

- **DON'T HANG OR TIE CLOTHESLINES, HAMMOCKS, AND EQUIPMENT ON OR TO TREES.** You may see this being commonly practiced In many developed campgrounds, but be responsible and do your part to reduce dam-age to trees and shrubs.

- **IF YOU TEND TO USE THE BATHROOM MULTIPLE TIMES AT NIGHT, PLAN AHEAD.** Leaving a warm sleeping bag and stumbling around in the dark to find the restroom—be it a pit toilet, a fully plumbed comfort station, or just the woods—is not fun. Keep a flashlight and any other accoutrements you may need by the tent door, and know exactly where to head in the dark.

- **WHEN YOU CAMP AT A DISPERSED SITE, KNOW HOW TO GO.** The lack of toilet facilities and water is the biggest challenge. Bringing large filled water jugs and a portable toilet are the easiest and most environmentally friendly solutions. A variety of portable toilets are available from outdoor-supply catalogs; in a pinch, a 5-gallon bucket fixed with a toilet seat and lined with a heavy-duty plastic trash bag will work just as well. (Be sure to pack out the trash bag.)

  A second, less desirable method is to dig 8-inch-deep catholes. These should be located at least 200 yards from campsites, trails, and water and in inconspicuous locations with as much undergrowth as possible. (Be creative and find spots with a great view—just make sure you aren't providing a great view for others!) Cover the hole with a thin layer of soil after each use, and *do not burn or bury your toilet paper*—pack it out in resealable plastic bags. If you'll be in the campsite for several days, dig a new hole each day, being careful to replace the topsoil over the hole from the day before.

  In addition to the plastic bags, your outdoor-toilet cache should include a garden trowel, toilet paper, and premoistened towelettes. Select a trowel with a well-designed handle that can also double as a toilet paper dispenser.

- **IF YOU AREN'T HIKING TO A PRIMITIVE CAMPSITE, DON'T SKIMP ON FOOD.** Plan tasty meals, and bring everything you'll need to prepare, cook, eat, and clean up. That said, don't duplicate equipment such as cooking pots among the members of your group. Carry what you need, but don't turn the trip into a cross-country moving experience.

- **KEEP A CLEAN KITCHEN AREA,** and avoid leaving food scraps on the ground both during and after your visit. Maintain a group trash bag, and be sure to secure it in your vehicle or a bearproof food locker at night. Many sites have a pack-in/pack-out rule, and that means everything: no cheating by tossing orange peels, eggshells, or apple cores in the shrubs.

- **DO YOUR PART TO HELP PREVENT BEARS FROM BECOMING CONDITIONED TO SEEKING HUMAN FOOD.** The constant search for food influences every aspect of a bear's life, so while camping in bear country, store food in your vehicle or in site-provided bearproof boxes. Keep food (including canned goods, soft drinks, and beer) and garbage secured, and resist the temptation to take food into your tent. You'll also need to stow scented or flavored toiletries such as toothpaste and lip balm, as well as cooking grease and pet food. Common sense and adherence to the simple rules posted at the campgrounds will help keep you and the bears safe and healthy. (See page 6 for what to do if you encounter a bear.)

- **USE ESTABLISHED FIRE RINGS, AND ALWAYS INQUIRE ABOUT CURRENT FIRE RESTRICTIONS.** Don't burn garbage in your campfire—trash often doesn't burn completely, and fire rings fill with burned litter over time. Be sure your fire is totally extinguished when you leave the area. If you cook with a Dutch oven, be sure to use a fire pan, and elevate it to avoid scorching or burning the ground.

Note that bringing your own firewood from home is frowned upon by many campground operators, so check ahead to see if it's allowed. Bringing in wood from outside of the area could introduce pests that are harmful to the forest, so if it's prohibited by the campground you plan to visit, use deadfall found near your campsite—again, only if permitted—or purchase wood at the camp store.

- **DON'T BATHE OR WASH DISHES AND LAUNDRY IN STREAMS AND LAKES.** Food scraps are unsightly and can be potentially harmful to fish, and even biodegradable soap can be harmful to fragile aquatic environments.

- **BE COURTEOUS TO OTHER CAMPERS.** Observe quiet hours, keep noise to a minimum, and keep pets leashed and under control.

- **MOST IMPORTANTLY, PLEASE LEAVE YOUR CAMP CLEANER THAN YOU FOUND IT.** Pick up all trash and microlitter in your site, including in your fire ring. Disperse leftover brush used for firewood.

Miner Lake *(see Miner Lake Campground, page 155)*

NORTHWEST MONTANA

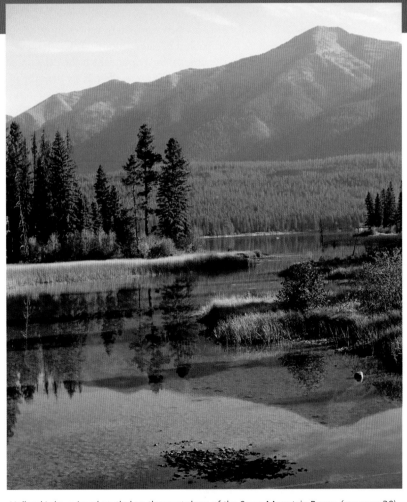

Holland Lake, a jewel nestled on the west slope of the Swan Mountain Range *(see page 30)*

⚠ Bad Medicine Campground

Beauty: ★★★★ / Privacy: ★★★★ / Quiet: ★★★★★ / Spaciousness: ★★★★★ / Security: ★★★★★ /
Cleanliness: ★★★★★

Nearby Ross Creek Cedars is as close as Montana gets to a rainforest.

Driving the densely forested access road to this campground provides a strong contrast to the dramatic peaks you see to the east along MT 56. Part of the 94,000-acre Cabinet Mountain Wilderness, these mountains top out at under 7,000 feet but seem to tower over the landscape. It's not an optical illusion. The fact that their base elevations are so low provides 4,000 feet of visible mountainside, making them just as impressive as the 10,000-foot peaks around Red Lodge.

In this peaceful setting on the southwest corner of Bull Lake, you'll find a variety of options under the conifer canopy. The well-spaced sites are level, and tents definitely rule the upper blufftop loop. The sites there are plentiful and spacious, and it's easy to orient your camp to create privacy. Sites 3, 4, and 12–15 are best for tenters, especially family groups.

That rapping noise you may hear is probably a pileated woodpecker. *Dryocopus pileatus,* for all you Woody Woodpecker fans, is the original bird upon which the cartoon character was based. If you want to look for these birds, try the large, old trees where they typically nest in jackhammered holes or snags formed in the treetops. Large, downed logs produce a feast of carpenter ants and beetle larvae, which are important to the woodpecker's diet.

Watch for other birds and wildlife, including red crossbill, pine siskin, and Steller's jay in the early morning, along with deer and an occasional elk. Coyote may be heard at night, but they tend to stay away from the campground area.

With 7 miles of lake beckoning, a canoe or boat might be a great addition to your gear, especially if you want to pursue the kokanee found in the deeper waters. If you don't have a boat, however, you can fish from the shore and try landing a largemouth bass or brook or rainbow trout. If the fish aren't biting, take a refreshing swim or relax on the shore. In general, this is a peaceful site, although on busy weekends there may be a bit too much boat noise during the day. But don't let that scare you away; this is still a wonderful campground.

Four miles away at Ross Creek Cedars Scenic Area is a unique cluster of old-growth timber spared from the loggers' saws. Views of the Cabinet Mountain

Loop trail in Ross Creek Cedars Scenic Area

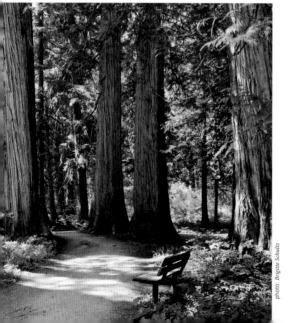

photo: *Brigitte Schultz*

Wilderness to the east are an extra delight on the narrow, winding road to the picnic area and parking lot of Ross Creek Cedars. You should make time to explore this U.S. Forest Service–designated scenic area. A mile-long loop trail with a wealth of interpretive signs winds along the base of massive, 175-foot-tall Western red cedars, some as old as 1,000 years. These ancient mammoths, up to 12 feet in diameter, dwarf the mature Western hemlocks, Western white pines, Western larches, mountain maples, and lodgepole pines that round out the forest.

The humid forest floor at Ross Creek Cedars, with its babbling streams, lush ferns, and variety of wildflowers, is as close as Montana gets to a rainforest. The cathedral hush is calming, and the minimal bugs (due to the altitude) are a pleasant surprise. Try finding some of the burned stumps throughout the forest. They are remnants of the August 1910 fire, during which a virtual hurricane of flames swept across the region, burning more than 3 million acres in Idaho and western Montana.

Ross Creek Cedars offers additional hiking options. Ross Creek Trail #142 is a 9-mile out-and-back hike to Sawtooth Mountain that follows the creek beneath a shelter of cedars and hemlocks. For those seeking a bit more exertion, Spar Peak Trail #324 is a 6.5-mile out-and-back from Spar Lake. Fire prompted a trail closure in 2007, but the trail was reopened in 2016. With a 3,000-foot altitude gain from the lake to Spar Peak, the view is worth it for those who can handle the trek.

You'll find a different view of the forest 10 miles south of the campground off MT 56, at the historic 1908 Bull River Guard Station. From MT 56, take Forest Service Road 407 east for 2 miles to FR 2278, then stay to the right and drive another mile to the parking area. This section of forest was impacted by the 1910 firestorm, so this provides an opportunity to see what a century of ecosystem regeneration looks like. The ranger station itself has been converted into a rental cabin equipped with bedding, an electric stove, basic furnishings, and an outdoor toilet, and can be booked online at recreation.gov.

Bad Medicine Campground

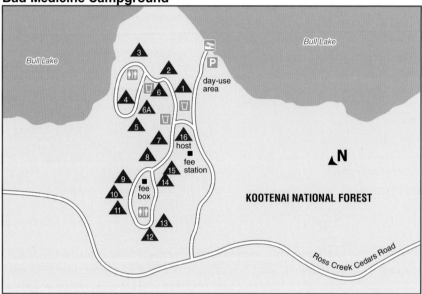

GETTING THERE

From Troy, take US 2 south 3 miles to the junction with MT 56. Turn right and go 21 miles south on MT 56 to Ross Creek Cedars Road, at the south end of Bull Lake. Turn right and follow signs for 2 miles to the campground.

From Trout Creek, take MT 200 north for 18 miles to MT 56. Turn right and go 15 miles north on MT 56 to Ross Creek Cedars Road, at the south end of Bull Lake. Turn left and follow signs for 2 miles to the campground.

GPS COORDINATES: N48° 9.260' W115° 52.167'

Big Arm Unit–Flathead Lake State Park Campground

Beauty: ★★★★ / Privacy: ★★★★ / Quiet: ★★★ / Spaciousness: ★★★★ / Security: ★★★★ / Cleanliness: ★★★★

These are the best tent sites on spectacular Flathead Lake.

Set between the Swan and Mission Ranges to the east and the Salish Mountains to the west, Flathead Lake is a sparkling northwestern Montana jewel carved thousands of years ago by receding glaciers. At 28 miles long, it's the largest freshwater lake west of the Mississippi and draws 80 percent of its water from a watershed larger than the states of Delaware and Rhode Island combined.

No wonder so many people drive up to Flathead, stopping at the highway stands selling Flathead cherries (try some—you won't be sorry). These prized cherries thrive on the microenvironment created by the lake. But visitors don't stop for long; they're on their way to a recreational heaven for boaters, anglers, swimmers, and just plain loafers.

However, a century ago things were not as bucolic—the timber industry was a strong presence, and the Flathead Indian Reservation was just being carved out. Back then it took 3–4 hours for steamboats to make the trip from north to south, and it could take longer depending on the weather. We're not sure which was more unpredictable, the weather or the Flathead Lake Monster.

The what? Yup, that's right, the Flathead Lake Monster was first seen by a group aboard a steamboat in 1889 who claimed they observed a 20-foot-long creature in the water. They weren't the only ones. Reported sightings have occurred in every decade since then. In 1955, someone claimed to have caught the monster. What they caught was actually a 181-pound white sturgeon now displayed in a museum in Polson. Here's the question: If the monster was caught, what do people keep seeing in the lake? In any case, it's a good sales pitch for

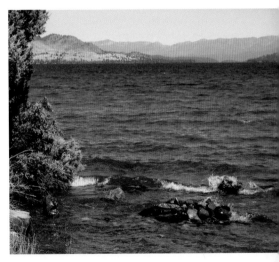

Flathead Lake is Montana's largest natural freshwater lake.

everything from hamburgers to T-shirts. But for some, the monster's legend is not all in jest. He (or she) still has some very serious believers.

There are six units of Flathead Lake State Park, with the Big Arm and Wild Horse Island Units being the two largest. Of the 41 campsites at Big Arm, the prime ones are right on the water. They might be a bit too close together, but claiming your own piece of Flathead Lake frontage outweighs a need for privacy.

KEY INFORMATION

ADDRESS: 28031 Big Arm State Park Road, Big Arm, MT 59910

CONTACT: 406-837-3041, stateparks.mt.gov /big-arm; reservations: reserveamerica.com

OPERATED BY: Big Arm Unit– Flathead Lake State Park

OPEN: Year-round when accessible; full services May–September

SITES: 41, plus 3 yurts

EACH SITE: Picnic table, fire ring

ASSIGNMENT: 10 sites are first come, first served; most sites are reservable.

REGISTRATION: At office; on-site self-registration when office is closed

FACILITIES: Hot showers, water spigots, flush toilets, boat ramp

PARKING: At campsites

FEE: $18 resident, $28 nonresident; $6/extra nonresident vehicle

ELEVATION: 2,953'

RESTRICTIONS:

Pets: On leash only

Fires: In fire rings only

Alcohol: Permitted

Vehicles: 40-foot length limit

Other: 14-day stay limit; firewood; tribal/ state fishing permits required

---

For a somewhat different tenting experience, consider renting one of the yurts at Big Arm. The yurt as a dwelling dates back at least 1,000 years, when it was used as a traditional home for Central Asian nomads, and its simple design is a masterpiece of geometric engineering. A round lattice frame forms the round wall, with roof beams leading to a smaller diameter roof ring to allow for light and ventilation. Two of the yurts at Big Arm sleep four people each, and a third sleeps six. They are complete with beds and tables.

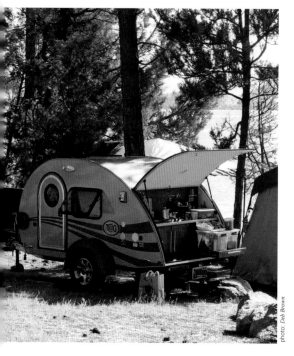

This state park has plentiful camping options.

photo: Deb Brown

Fishing from shore or boat is productive for whitefish or lake trout, while yellow perch are found only at the southern end of the lake near Big Arm. This end of the lake is on the Flathead Indian Reservation, so you need both a state fishing license and a tribal fishing permit. Regulations, licenses, charter trips, and boat rentals are available in Big Arm and Polson.

This campground is also one of the best locations from which to launch an exploration of Wild Horse Island. Accessible only by boat, this island fills 2,163 acres of Flathead Lake. You'll find a magnificent and diverse collection of wildlife and native plants here. Along with the small namesake herd of wild horses, you may encounter bighorn sheep, eagles, osprey, mule deer, songbirds, geese, owls, and a variety of small mammals. Bring plenty of water, since there is no drinking water available. There is a composting toilet on the island.

If you're seeking a little more challenge, try the Flathead Lake marine trail. This "trail" is actually a collection of islands and other points around the lake that can be accessed by sea kayak. Maps and brochures detail the specifics of the lake's more than 128 miles of shoreline. You can easily design a day trip between nearby sites or plan a week-long excursion. Less experienced paddlers should stay closer to shore, and those crossing the lake are warned that a calm morning can shift to wicked winds and 5-foot waves very quickly.

Big Arm Unit–Flathead Lake State Park Campground

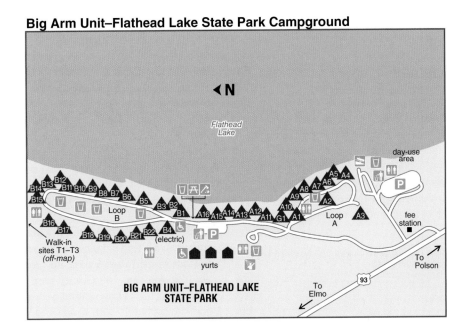

GETTING THERE

From Polson, take US 93 north for 14 miles to the campground entrance, on the right.

GPS COORDINATES: N47° 48.798' W114° 18.924'

3

⛺ Big Creek Campground

Beauty: ★★★★ / Privacy: ★★★ / Quiet: ★★★★ / Spaciousness: ★★★★ / Security: ★★★★★ / Cleanliness: ★★★★★

Big Creek sits on the banks of the wild and scenic North Fork at the front door of Glacier National Park.

Big Creek sits on the banks of the Flathead River's North Fork, at the front door of Glacier National Park. Flowing along and defining the park's western boundary, the North Fork is one of Montana's premier rivers and in 1976 was designated a part of the National Wild and Scenic River System from the Canadian border to its confluence with the Middle Fork.

At the campground, the sites are set among lodgepole pines, and the rushing waters of the North Fork can be heard everywhere. The best sites are 5–15, because they back up to the river and have plenty of space between them. If these aren't available, sites 16, 17, and 19–22 also have a fair amount of privacy, since they are on the outside loop with no other sites behind them. Site 22 sits even farther apart on a slight rise overlooking a large, open field.

In August 2001, a lightning strike started the 71,000-acre Moose Fire, which burned right through this campground. Fortunately, conditions at the time mitigated the damage, and the fire burned little of the crown cover. Ground-cover vegetation, however, was affected and is slowly making a comeback. You'll see the regeneration for yourself as the new plants fill in space between you and your neighbors. Fire visited again in 2003 when the Robert Fire burned much of the area south of the campground.

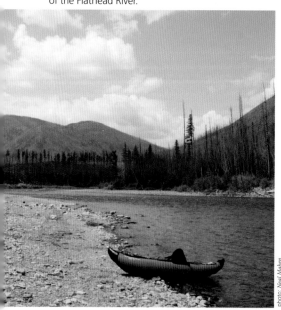

Paddling dreams come true on the North Fork of the Flathead River.

photo: Neal Maben

Because the campground has just 21 sites, you may find it difficult to get a spot in midsummer after 6 p.m., so reserve ahead if you can. The Glacier area gets more than 1.5 million visitors each year, and campgrounds both inside and outside of the park tend to fill up fast. If you haven't reserved and you wait until late in the day to set up camp, it may be challenging to find a site anywhere.

Big Creek is busy in the summer. The day-use area is crowded even during the week, and the adjacent Glacier Institute is a nonprofit organization offering a full range of educational classes, workshops, and field trips for kids and adults. In addition, Big Creek is a popular put-in and takeout for rafters and floaters.

Note: At press time in 2017, boating was prohibited in Glacier due to detection of invasive mussel, so call or check online for the latest information.

KEY INFORMATION

ADDRESS: North Fork Road, Columbia Falls, MT 59912

CONTACT: 406-387-3800, www.fs.usda.gov /flathead; reservations: 877-444-6777, recreation.gov

OPERATED BY: Flathead National Forest, Tally Lake Ranger District

OPEN: Memorial Day weekend–Labor Day

SITES: 21, plus 1 group site

EACH SITE: Picnic table, fire grate

ASSIGNMENT: First come, first served or by reservation

REGISTRATION: On-site self-registration or online

FACILITIES: Hand-pump well, vault toilets, boat launch (but see below), day-use area

PARKING: At campsites

FEE: $14

ELEVATION: 3,300'

RESTRICTIONS:

Pets: On leash only

Fires: In fire rings only

Alcohol: Permitted

Vehicles: 40-foot length limit

Other: 16-day stay limit; bear-country food storage restrictions. No boating in Glacier at press time; call/ check online for the latest information.

Independent and guided floating on the North Fork is very popular, and the 18-mile section between Polebridge and Big Creek is easiest for novices once the spring runoff has ended, usually by July. This section is also less crowded, since more experienced floaters generally head for the 8-mile whitewater section running south of the campground to the Glacier Rim takeout.

Many fish and wildlife species can be found at the point where Big Creek drains into the North Fork. The river provides cold, clear, fast-moving water, which is vital to sustaining the native bull trout (*Salvelinus confluentus*) as it ascends the North and Middle Forks of the Flathead River to seek out smaller tributary streams and creeks in which to spawn. These strikingly colorful fish are also known by the name Dolly Varden. If you've brushed up on your Charles Dickens, you may remember the book *Barnaby Rudge* and the character Dolly Varden, who, like the bull trout, dressed quite colorfully in flashes of green with pink polka dots. The bull trout is federally listed as a threatened species, and the state of Montana has been aggressively managing those found here to ensure that the population does not further decline and move from threatened to endangered. These efforts have been successful to the point that regulations have been relaxed in some waterways, but, as always, be familiar with current regulations before you wet your hook.

The fairly difficult Glacier View Mountain Trail #381 begins at the campground trail-head and is an 8-mile round-trip that gains nearly 3,000 feet in elevation ascending the mountain peak. From there, Demers Ridge Trail #266 continues another 4 miles to Outside North Fork Road (Forest Service Road 486) near the Camas Creek entrance to Glacier. Both trails offer excellent views of Glacier and the North Fork area. Trailheads for the 17-mile Ralph Thayer Memorial National Recreation Trail and the 10-mile Smoky Range National Recreation Trail are within driving distance. Additional information and maps can be obtained from the ranger district headquarters.

The closest hike in Glacier begins near the Camas Creek entrance. This 6-mile round-trip to Huckleberry Lookout traverses an area partially burned in the 2001 Moose Fire, but there are pockets that haven't burned since the 1967 fire. These pockets are maturing and provide an educational contrast to the land you'll encounter at Big Creek and elsewhere on your hike. The trail takes you along the creek and up some steep slopes before hitting the ridge, where you'll be above the tree line. Wildflowers dazzle here all summer, especially through the first mile or so. More than 200 bird species have been seen in the North Fork area, so maybe you'll be one of the lucky visitors who get a glimpse of a great gray owl or a Le Conte's sparrow.

Big Creek Campground

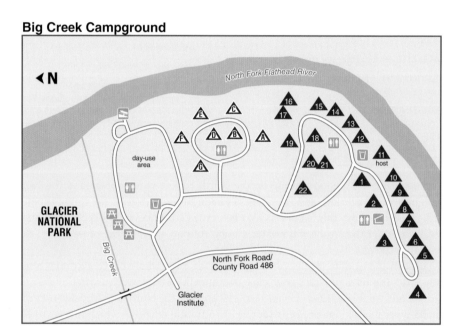

GETTING THERE

From Columbia Falls, take North Fork Road (County Road 486) north for 20.5 miles to the campground. The road turns to dirt after 12.5 miles.

GPS COORDINATES: N48° 35.939' W114° 9.820'

4

Big Therriault Lake Campground

Beauty: ★★★★★ / Privacy: ★★★★★ / Quiet: ★★★★★ / Spaciousness: ★★★★ / Security: ★★★★★ / Cleanliness: ★★★★★

Big Therriault wins the prize for "most off the beaten path."

Of all the campgrounds selected, this one wins the prize for "most off the beaten path." On the drive in, you may feel you are on a dull, desolate road leading nowhere. But hang in there—you will be rewarded. As the road climbs, a few more trees appear, and then suddenly you'll arrive in a thick pine and spruce forest on the clearest, most pristine mountain lake you've ever seen without a backpack. You'll be only a few miles from Canada and will have more bears for neighbors than people.

The campground itself is small, only 5 acres, and the sites are set on a hillside around a single loop with plenty of understory for privacy. Most sites are suited for tents, although the two pull-through spots are better left for RVs. None of the sites sit directly on the lake, and there aren't any with clear views due to the thick forest, but most are adjacent to the 1-mile trail around the lake. This trail provides a short course in glacial geology; you will see grooves carved by the glaciers and moraines formed by the debris left behind.

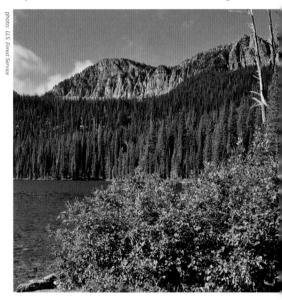

photo: U.S. Forest Service

The highlights of the trail include wildflower-strewn meadows and a variety of wildlife: deer, elk, osprey, eagles, the occasional mountain lion, and, if you're extremely lucky, a wolverine. Centered within the loop is a 55-acre lake with a multihued rock bottom and a wealth of cutthroat trout. An afternoon spent paddling a canoe or kayak in this serene spot is an ideal antidote for the tension of everyday life. In the morning you'll awaken to songbirds, and in the evening you'll hear the calls of loons.

View along Big Therriault Lake

Just down the road is Little Therriault Lake Campground, with six roomy and secluded campsites. This lake is smaller (28 acres), but you'll find a lakeside trail here as well. At the north end of the lake is a trailhead into the Ten Lakes Scenic Area, where hikers and horses are allowed but ATVs are not.

While not an officially designated wilderness area, this 34,000-acre, unspoiled slice of roadless land extends to the Canadian border and is managed by Kootenai National Forest. Prehistoric glaciers carved the deep cirques and rocky basins that ultimately became alpine lakes. The waters are spectacularly clear, wildflowers bloom profusely, and huckleberries are

KEY INFORMATION

ADDRESS: Therriault Lakes Road
(Forest Road 319), Eureka, MT 59917

CONTACT: 406-296-2536; www.fs.usda.gov
/kootenai

OPERATED BY: Kootenai National Forest,
Fortine Ranger District

OPEN: July–Labor Day (may be open earlier or
later if weather allows, possibly without
water or fees)

SITES: 9

EACH SITE: Picnic table, fire grate, bear-
resistant box

ASSIGNMENT: First come, first served;
no reservations

REGISTRATION: On-site self-registration

FACILITIES: Hand-pump well, vault toilets,
carry-in boat launch

PARKING: At campsites

FEE: $5

ELEVATION: 5,554'

RESTRICTIONS:

Pets: On leash only

Fires: In fire rings only

Alcohol: Permitted

Vehicles: 32-foot length limit

Other: 16-day stay limit; bear-country
food storage restrictions; pack in,
pack out

abundant for those who keep their eyes open. Waterfalls appear unexpectedly, and you can literally hike all day without seeing anyone else.

A day-hike loop leaves from the south end of Big Therriault Lake, heads over Therriault Pass, winds along the Highline Trail and St. Clair Peak, and ends at the south end of Little Therriault Lake. This route takes you up about 1,500 feet and provides dramatic vistas across the Whitefish Range into Canada. From the same trailhead, you can take Highline Trail left for a hike to the summit of Stahl Peak. The view from this lookout is to the south, where you'll have a pretty good chance of seeing bighorn sheep along the mountainsides throughout the summer months.

From the trailhead northwest of Little Therriault Lake, you can take the 5-mile out-and-back hike to Bluebird Lake. Elevation gain on this hike is less than 1,000 feet, and you won't encounter any super-steep or difficult sections. If you start early enough, you can spend a relaxing day at the lake before heading back. A longer option is to continue past Bluebird Lake to Wolverine Lakes. You can make this hike either a 9-mile out-and-back or an 11.5-mile loop. The loop option brings you back on Tie Thru Trail #82; it is best spread over two or three days and is one of only several combinations that take hikers deep into this lush backcountry.

Stocking up on supplies, topping off the gas tank, and checking the air in your spare while passing through Eureka is a prudent idea. It's 36 long, bumpy miles to the campground. Cell phone reception is nonexistent, bears don't make the best auto mechanics, and if you get a yearning for a cold glass of milk, a nice juicy orange, or a super-gooey s'more, it will take you at least half the day to satisfy your craving. Wouldn't you rather be out hiking or just sitting by the lake enjoying the peace and quiet?

Big Therriault Lake Campground

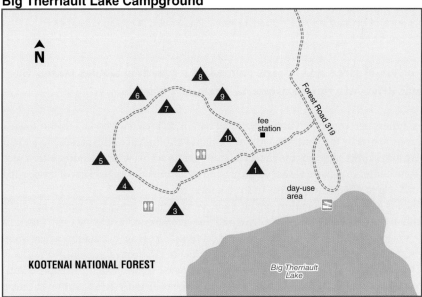

GETTING THERE

From Fortine, take US 93 northwest 3 miles. Turn right on Grave Creek Road (Forest Road 114) and go 12 miles to Therriault Lakes Road (FR 319). Continue straight on Therriault Lakes Road and follow signs for 16 miles to the campground. Therriault Lakes Road is a narrow, winding dirt road that requires patience.

GPS COORDINATES: N48° 56.177' W114° 52.686'

5

⛺ Cut Bank Campground

Beauty: ★★★★★ / Privacy: ★★★★★ / Quiet: ★★★★★ / Spaciousness: ★★★ / Security: ★★★ /
Cleanliness: ★★★★★

A mixture of pines and aspens painted on a mountain canvas makes the 5-mile drive into this campground a relaxing treat.

The southeastern corner of Glacier National Park is an area few people see, but those who do are surprised by the contrast with the verdant western half of the park, where the thick undergrowth often obscures the spectacular mountain scenery. In the southeastern section, you'll encounter expansive views, scrub ground cover mixed with pockets of trees, and lush riparian edges. The scenery seems to stretch forever.

Such is life from the comfort of Cut Bank. A mixture of pines and aspens painted on a mountain canvas makes the 5-mile drive into this campground a relaxing treat. Open-range cattle graze both sides of the road, so drive cautiously to avoid a situation where your car will be the loser. (In Montana, we don't fence cattle in—we fence them out.)

The campground is small, and RVs are discouraged from making the trip, so you will probably be sharing space only with nylon neighbors. Choose from 14 gravel tent pads framed in wood timbers—which serve as further evidence that RVers should keep looking. A mixture of fir, aspen, cottonwood, and ponderosa pine provides shade in this otherwise exposed area. Although the sites are fairly close together, each one offers enough space to make you feel like it's your own private piece of Glacier. In keeping with the wilderness theme, restrooms are rustic wood, not concrete, with one hole each. Bearproof food-storage boxes remind you to be conscientious and practice bear-aware camping techniques.

Tent site with a gorgeous Glacier view

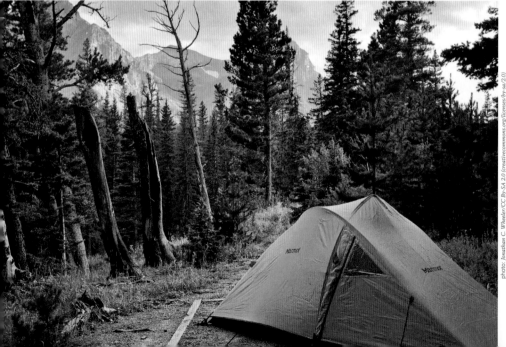

KEY INFORMATION

ADDRESS: North Fork Cut Bank Creek off MT 89, West Glacier, MT 59936

CONTACT: 406-888-7800, nps.gov/glac

OPERATED BY: Glacier National Park

OPEN: June–September

SITES: 14

EACH SITE: Picnic table, fire grate

ASSIGNMENT: First come, first served; no reservations

REGISTRATION: On-site self-registration

FACILITIES: Vault toilets; no drinking water available

PARKING: At campsites

FEE: $10

ELEVATION: 5,500'

RESTRICTIONS:

Pets: On leash only

Fires: In fire rings only

Alcohol: Permitted

Vehicles: 22-foot length limit

Other: 14-day stay limit; bear-country food storage restrictions. No boating in Glacier at press time; call/check online for the latest information.

Additional information is stapled to picnic tables, and park staff patrols the area, just in case you need help remembering.

Sites 8 and 10 on the outside loop are the most desirable, with lots of room and the most privacy. Site 11 is roomy as well but isn't as private, since it adjoins the host's site. Overall, it's a quiet area with most people out on the trails during the day. Since it stays light until around 10 p.m. in summer, you can enjoy plenty of peaceful downtime even if you just hang out around camp. Early morning and dusk are the best times to view wildlife such as black and grizzly bears, deer, and elusive wolves, but eagles and hawks can be seen anytime. Check with the ranger station for current high-activity areas.

Fishing for brook and rainbow trout or mountain whitefish in the North Fork of Cut Bank Creek wiles away the hours for many, while others rise to the challenge of hiking from the trailhead. There are several options, but for the first 4 miles, all follow the same route through meadows along the creek before beginning to gradually climb. At the junction near Atlantic Creek, the left fork takes you 2.6 miles to Medicine Grizzly Peak (8,315') and its waterfalls and then on to Morningstar Lake. From there it's a steep 3-mile climb (quite possibly through snowfields) to Katoya and Pitamakan Lakes and Pitamakan Pass. Along the way, you'll see Red Mountain (9,389') to the east and Mount Phillips (9,627') to the southwest.

Note: At press time in 2017, boating was prohibited in Glacier due to detection of invasive mussel, so call or check online for the latest information.

Choose to veer right at the junction, and in 0.5 mile you'll have another decision: Medicine Grizzly Lake or Triple Divide Pass. Many people do both, because it's only 1.5 miles to the lake and 2.5 miles to the pass, but this requires a pretty early start. The 14.4-mile round-trip hike to the pass is a gradual climb without steep pitches or switchbacks, and views are continuous. This hike also brings you to the base of Triple Divide Peak (8,020'), a unique geographic location where a three-sided glacial horn formed as separate glaciers eroded the mountain's sides. The result is that water or snow collecting on the northeast side drains into the Saskatchewan River, Hudson Bay, and then the Arctic Ocean; water on the west side drains into Flathead River, Clark Fork River, and on into the Columbia River and Pacific

Ocean. From the south side, water makes its way to the Missouri River via Atlantic Creek and Marias River and then on into the Mississippi River and Gulf of Mexico.

On these trails you'll encounter plenty of wildflowers and wildlife, along with an ever-changing assortment of rain, snow, sunshine, and hail. Be prepared, be aware, and have fun.

Cut Bank Campground

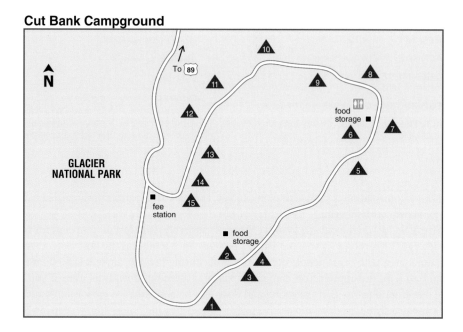

GETTING THERE

From St. Mary, take US 89 south for 15 miles to the park entrance road. Turn right and go west for 5 miles to the campground.

From East Glacier Park, take MT 49 north for 11.8 miles to US 89. Continue north on US 89 for 5 miles to the park entrance road. Turn left and go west for 5 miles to the campground. MT 49, a narrow, winding road with a 21-foot vehicle-length restriction, requires caution and patience. As an alternative, you can take US 2 east 12 miles from East Glacier Park to US 89 and then proceed 17 miles north on US 89 to the park entrance road.

GPS COORDINATES: N48° 36.109' W113° 23.019'

6

Fish Creek Campground

Beauty: ★★★★★ / Privacy: ★★★★ / Quiet: ★★★★ / Spaciousness: ★★★★ / Security: ★★★★★ /
Cleanliness: ★★★★★

Smack in the middle of the 2003 Robert Fire, Fish Creek emerged unscathed.

Although you'd never know it by looking at the fir forest immediately surrounding it, this campground was smack in the middle of the 39,000-acre Robert Fire of 2003. Only through aggressive suppression activity were crews able to protect this pocket of Glacier National Park during the fiery onslaughts.

On the drive to the campground from the park entrance, about one-half mile past the Apgar area, you'll see Bullhead Lodge on the shore of Lake McDonald. The lodge once served as artist Charlie Russell's private home. Private homes were common in the park's early days, but only a few are left, and they aren't for sale. They remain only because they've been in the same families for a long time.

As one of only two campgrounds at Glacier accepting reservations (the other is St. Mary), Fish Creek, surprisingly, rarely fills up, even during July and early August. Three of the four loops (B, C, and D) sit between Fish Creek and Lake McDonald, but few sites have clear water views due to the dense forest. That's OK, since the trees provide more privacy than you'd expect at such a large campground.

None of the sites on Loop A stand out as exceptional, but most are well suited for tents. The most coveted sites on Loop B are the odd-numbered sites that lie along the loop's south side. Sites

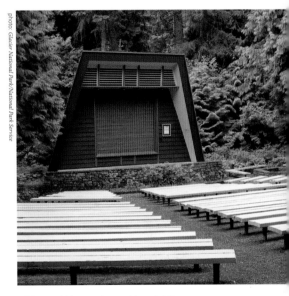

photo *Glacier National Park/National Park Service*

This amphitheater is used for nightly ranger programs.

42 and 43 are nice as well, but they're opposite the restrooms and path to loop C. Sites 47 and 49 offer a unique option—both are raised and require a bit more energy to set up camp, but it's definitely worth the effort for the sense of privacy. Loop C provides spectacular lake views from sites 106, 108, and 110. Site 150, on the connecting road between loops C and D, is the most private. This site, along with sites 173 and 174, has the best lake views, but all three are tough to get and very popular with RVs.

Due to restrictions that protect the habitat of nesting Harlequin ducks, Fish Creek is one of the park's tributaries where fishing is not allowed. But feel free to visit the creek and the ducks. You might even try braving the chilly waters to wade a bit.

KEY INFORMATION

ADDRESS: Camas Road, West Glacier, MT 59936

CONTACT: 406-888-7800, nps.gov/glac; reservations: 877-444-6777, recreation.gov

OPERATED BY: Glacier National Park

OPEN: Mid-June–early September

SITES: 178

EACH SITE: Picnic table, fire grate

ASSIGNMENT: First come, first served or by reservation

REGISTRATION: On-site self-registration or online

FACILITIES: Water spigots, flush toilets, dump station, amphitheater, interpretive activities and programs

PARKING: At campsites

FEE: $23

ELEVATION: 3,150'

RESTRICTIONS:

Pets: On leash only, not permitted on trails or along lakeshores

Fires: In fire rings only

Alcohol: Permitted

Vehicles: 35-foot length limit; 2 vehicles/site

Other: 14-day stay limit July–Labor Day and 30-day limit the rest of the year; bear-country food storage restrictions; no firearms; no firewood gathering; special fishing regulations. No boating in Glacier at press time; call/check online for the latest information.

Note: At press time in 2017, boating was prohibited in Glacier due to detection of invasive mussel, so call or check online for the latest information.

A hike along the northern shore of Lake McDonald gives you an up-close view of the fire damage along with the regrowth already transforming the devastation. This trail is 6.6 gentle miles from end to end with several lakeshore overlooks. Fishing along the shoreline is easy, and no license is required to pursue the cutthroat, rainbow, and lake trout. Early morning and early evening, when the wind is calm, are the best times for fishing the clear, cold water of this glacial lake.

An easy hike to Rocky Point begins near the campground, and dozens more hiking trails exist throughout the park. A few miles north, on Camas Road, is the trailhead for the Huckleberry Mountain Trails—a level 0.9-mile interpretive trail and a 6-mile out-and-back trail to a manned lookout. Ultimately, it will come down to a question of time and stamina. Obtain a trail guide and be prepared to have trouble choosing from the wealth of options, which range from quick jaunts to multiday backpacking trips.

Nightly amphitheater programs explain the park's flora and fauna and provide historical anecdotes and insight into the weather patterns. Questions are welcome, and the discussion often extends well into the evening. Rangers also lead hikes along Huckleberry Nature Trail to observe the regeneration occurring after various fires.

More options are available at nearby Apgar, where programs are held at the amphitheater four nights a week. At the Discovery Center, visitors can explore hands-on exhibits about the park's natural residents and geological creation. Food service, gift shops, and basic supplies are also available at Apgar.

Fish Creek Campground A

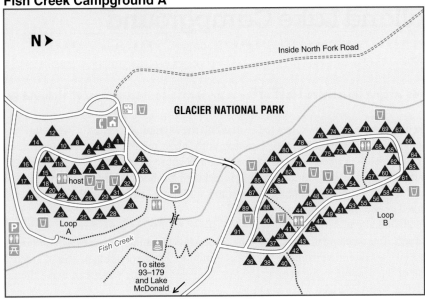

Fish Creek Campground B

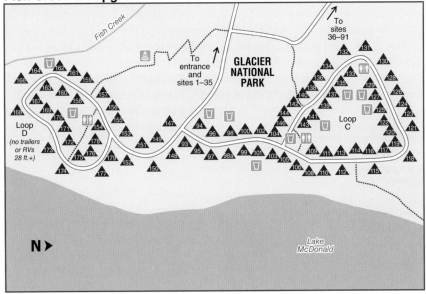

GETTING THERE

From the West Glacier entrance to Glacier National Park, take the park road 2 miles north to Camas Road. Turn left and go northwest for 2 miles to the campground entrance, on the right. Follow Fish Creek Campground Road for about a mile to the campground.

GPS COORDINATES: N48° 32.867' W113° 59.117'

7

Holland Lake Campground

Beauty: ★★★★★ / Privacy: ★★★★ / Quiet: ★★★★ / Spaciousness: ★★★★ / Security: ★★★★ / Cleanliness: ★★★★

Sites atop a lakeshore bluff offer a dramatic postcard view of Holland Falls.

Tucked between the Swan Range to the east and the Mission Range to the west, the Seeley-Swan Valley is a popular outdoor paradise with lakes, mountains, rivers, small streams, and trails. Visitors can enjoy the best that Mother Nature has to offer year-round. You may wonder why a place that sounds this busy is included in a book where the idea is to get away from it all. It's simple: the setting is awesome, and, especially during the week, it isn't as crowded as you might expect.

Holland Lake was formed when the last glacial ice melted from this area some 10,000 years ago. The receding glaciers deposited sediments, forming moraines, which now hold back a lake fed by runoff from the spectacular mountains surrounding it. This 427-acre lake is one of the deepest in the area at 155 feet. The clarity of the water can make the depth deceiving, so be prepared when boating.

Campsites here are in two loops, and the very best sites (1, 2, and 6) lie in the Larch Loop, which is the first loop off the entrance road. Sitting atop a lakeshore bluff, these sites offer a dramatic postcard view of Holland Falls. You'll also get a nice view from sites 3 and 5 but will be close to the restroom and trash dumpster. The sites here have less understory than those on the Bay Loop, but they're large, with plenty of space for pitching a tent, and uneven sites have gravel tent pads.

The best sites on the Bay Loop are 18 and 30, right on the lake, although you may consider this loop less desirable since it attracts more RVs. It also puts you closer to Holland Lake Lodge and its activity, although the lodge's rustic bar and dining room are a draw for many visitors.

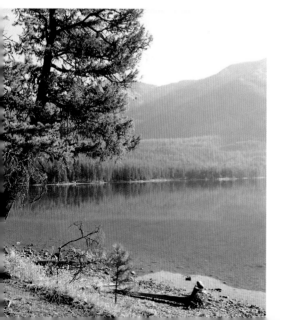

Holland Lake affords fishing, swimming, camping, and wilderness access.

If you bring a boat, head for deeper waters to find kokanee, but not during prime weekend hours when motorboats and Jet Skis may be overwhelming. Fishing from shore is quieter and yields perch, cutthroat, and rainbow trout. Just be sure you know how to identify a bull trout so you don't mistake it for a cutthroat and end up with a hefty fine. Bull trout are currently protected in Montana, and you'll be preventing the species from reproducing by frying one up for dinner.

On a hot day, try a swim in the crystalline lake. But even in late July it may be too cold for comfort. Less hearty souls are content to seek out a nice spot along

KEY INFORMATION

ADDRESS: Holland Lake Road, Condon, MT 59826

CONTACT: 406-837-7500, www.fs.usda.gov /flathead; reservations: 877-444-6777, recreation.gov

OPERATED BY: Flathead National Forest, Swan Lake Ranger District

OPEN: Mid-May–September

SITES: 39

EACH SITE: Picnic table, fire grate

ASSIGNMENT: First come, first served and by reservation

REGISTRATION: On-site self-registration or online

FACILITIES: Water spigots, flush and vault toilets, boat ramp, beach, dump station

PARKING: At campsites

FEE: $15

ELEVATION: 4,050'

RESTRICTIONS:

Pets: On leash only

Fires: In fire rings only

Alcohol: Permitted

Vehicles: 50-foot length limit

Other: 16-day stay limit; bear-country food-storage requirements

---

the shoreline to wade and enjoy the mirrored image of the Swan Range peaks or to take the 0.6-mile nature trail along the shore. Elk and deer frequent the lakeshore, and an occasional bear shows up to keep things interesting.

No visit to Holland Lake is complete without a hike to Holland Falls at the base of the Swan Range. This 3.5-mile hike is along National Recreation Trail #416, which begins at the north end of the lake and climbs steadily to the 40-foot falls and a spectacular view of the Swan Valley and the Mission Mountains. You'll find several natural nooks and crannies along the way for picnics and just enjoying the day. It's a popular trail on weekends, so early-morning treks are best for campers seeking solitude. In addition, bugs can be fierce along the trail, especially after it rains.

If you still have energy, this trail continues on as the Upper Holland Loop, a fairly strenuous additional 10 miles that climb 3,000 feet to Upper Holland Lake and Sapphire Lake on the edge of the Bob Marshall Wilderness before returning to the falls. From this loop, you can hike spurs to the Holland Lookout, Necklace Lakes chains, Big Salmon Lake, and Gordon Pass. Except on the trail to the falls, you'll be sharing the path with horses, but motorized vehicles and bikes are prohibited.

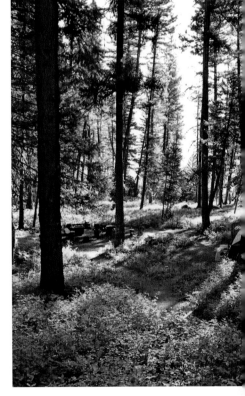

All sites at Holland Lake are near the lake and lie under forest canopy.

Holland Lake Campground

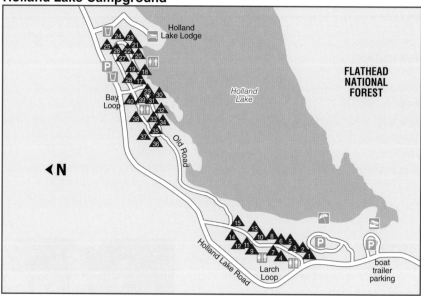

GETTING THERE

From Condon, take MT 83 southeast to highway marker 35.5. Turn left and go east 3 miles on Holland Lake Road (Forest Service Road 44) to the campground.

From Seeley Lake, take MT 83 northeast for 20 miles to highway marker 35.5. Turn right and go east for 3 miles on Holland Lake Road (FR 44) to the campground.

GPS COORDINATES: N47° 26.779' W113° 36.000'

8

Kintla Lake Campground

Beauty: ★★★★★ / Privacy: ★★★★ / Quiet: ★★★★★ / Spaciousness: ★★★★ / Security: ★★★★★ / Cleanliness: ★★★★★

Camp near an isolated mountain lake at the base of towering, snowcapped mountains.

Driving the Inside North Fork Road to Kintla Lake offers an excellent chance to view wildlife, wildflowers, and the rebirth of Glacier after the fires of 1988 and 2003. But getting here isn't easy. You won't need four-wheel drive, but the road is extremely rough, and you should plan on averaging 15 mph. This was the first road in the area, developed by oil barons in the early 1900s as they began drilling near Kintla Lake. Things were going well (no pun intended) until they hit a gas vein, causing the whole operation to explode into flames. Meanwhile, the area was already on track for designation as a national park. When Glacier became the country's 10th national park in 1910, oil exploration ended, but drilling on the Rocky Mountain front and on land adjoining the park remains a divisive issue today.

Kintla is off the main track for Glacier's typical drive-through visitors, who often don't realize this region exists. But if you like isolated lakes at the base of towering, snowcapped mountains where deer, elk, and black bears are abundant and eagles are frequent visitors, this is a prime choice. The campsites themselves are not very private, since much of the understory was removed as a fire precaution, but the splendid location and potential for being one of the few people here are distinct advantages that more than offset the lack of screening. Sites here are similar to one another, with none actually situated on the lake, although sites 9–11 sit along the creek that runs between the lake and North Fork Flathead River.

The trailer near the lake is actually a ranger station that is infrequently staffed,

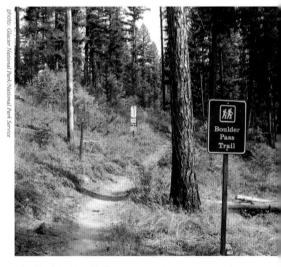

photo: *Glacier National Park/National Park Service*

The Boulder Pass Trail starts near the campground.

another indication that camping here requires preparation and self-reliance. The weather can be unpredictable—yes, it has snowed in every month of the year—and it's 15 miles to limited services in Polebridge. Cell phones probably won't work, no matter what your provider tells you, and you need to take the food storage restrictions seriously.

Fishing on the 8-mile-long lake, either from shore or from a canoe, is good for cutthroat trout and whitefish. If you're planning to wade or use a float tube, wearing insulated gear is essential since the water is always cold.

KEY INFORMATION

ADDRESS: Inside North Fork Road, West Glacier, MT 59936

CONTACT: 406-888-7800, nps.gov/glac

OPERATED BY: Glacier National Park

OPEN: Summer season, early June–early September; primitive season, mid-May–early June and early September–October 31. Call or check online for the latest information.

SITES: 13 tent sites

EACH SITE: Picnic table, fire grate

ASSIGNMENT: First come, first served; no reservations

REGISTRATION: On-site self-registration

FACILITIES: Hand-pump well, vault toilets

PARKING: At campsites

FEE: $15

ELEVATION: 4,008'

RESTRICTIONS:

Pets: On leash only, not permitted on trails or along lakeshore

Fires: In fire rings only

Alcohol: Permitted

Vehicles: RVs not recommended, 2 vehicles/site

Other: 14-day stay limit July–Labor Day and 30-day limit the rest of the year; bear-country food storage restrictions; no firearms; no firewood gathering; special fishing regulations. No boating in Glacier at press time; call/check online for the latest information.

Note: At press time in 2017, boating was prohibited in Glacier due to detection of invasive mussel, so call or check online for the latest information.

Hiking trails fan out along the shore and lead to backcountry sites on Upper Kintla Lake. Dramatic views of forested peaks along the northern shore contrast with those of the lake's southern shore, which were devastated in the 2003 Wedge Canyon fire. The campground itself was miraculously spared even though the fire burned 53,000 acres over a period of two months. About 2 miles from the campground, on Inside North Fork Road, is the trailhead for Kishenehn Creek Trail. This easy 4-mile trail includes two creek crossings and an excellent chance to see elk, moose, and maybe even a bear. Whenever hiking in Glacier, be sure you understand and follow safety precautions. They aren't tough or complicated, but they will help you have a safe and enjoyable hike.

If you're seeking a bit of civilization, it's about an hour by car to the hamlet of Polebridge. This tiny enclave is the stalwart heart of the North Fork region. Threatened by the Red Bench fire in 1988 and essentially shut down during the 2003 fire season, it has survived. Folks here are tough, resilient, and creative at keeping their community and way of life alive. Whether it's world-class music festivals or holiday celebrations, Polebridge attracts an eclectic mix of visitors and locals. A stop here is not complete without sampling the baked goods at the Polebridge Mercantile and reading the well-preserved news clippings that tell the area's history. Sit on the porch of this building, listed on the National Register of Historic Places, sip a cool drink, and plan the next phase of your visit to Glacier. If you've brought your mountain bike, the ride to Polebridge is a fairly level 29-mile round-trip. It can be a dusty ride at times but is an excellent opportunity for wildlife viewing, which just isn't possible when you're driving.

Another biking option is Hornet Peak Loop, which begins just north of Polebridge on Outside North Fork Road. This is a 21.5-mile ride (with a 1-mile spur trail you can hike to the lookout) along the southern edge of the area burned by the Wedge Canyon fire. The ride up is tough, with an elevation gain of more than 2,000 feet, but the descent will literally take your breath away.

Kintla Lake Campground

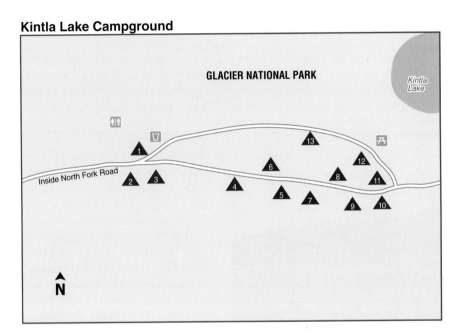

GETTING THERE

From West Glacier, take Camas Road 17 miles north to North Fork Road, and turn right. After 12.9 miles, turn right on Polebridge Loop. In 0.3 mile, turn left (north) on Glacier Drive and drive 1.4 miles. After crossing the North Fork Flathead River, turn left, with the Polebridge Ranger Station on your right, and make another left just past the ranger station onto Inside North Fork Road. In 4 miles, veer left and then right to continue north on Inside North Fork Road. Follow the road 10.2 miles farther to its dead end at Kintla Lake; the campground is at the end of the road.

GPS COORDINATES: N48° 56.155' W114° 20.843'

9

Lake Alva Campground

Beauty: ★★★★ / Privacy: ★★★★★ / Quiet: ★★★★ / Spaciousness: ★★★★ / Security: ★★★★★ /
Cleanliness: ★★★★★

Lake Alva is a gentle, wooded pearl where the haunting calls of loons echo through the night.

Along this stretch of the Clearwater River is a chain of lakes nestled in the valley like a string of pearls, each with its own unique features and characteristics. Lake Alva is a gentle, wooded pearl where the campsites are divided between two loops, with a third loop on the lake reserved for groups. The sites are well spaced and among the most private to be found at a developed campground.

Larch, fir, and alder trees anchor the screening between most sites. These trees buffer so well that even if a large RV is on the adjacent site, you probably won't know it. Each site is different, but sites 27, 37, 38, and 40 on the northern loop are the most private, with plenty of room for tents.

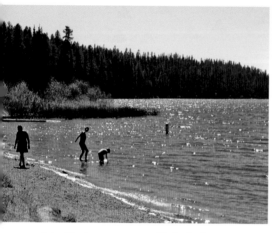

Lake Alva is synonymous with family fun.

The haunting calls of common loons echo throughout the day and into the night here, adding to the sense of wilderness even though you're not far from the highway. If you're lucky, you'll see them dive far beneath the surface and stay under water for long periods of time, using their daggerlike beaks to ferret out food.

The day-use area is busy on weekends and provides a boat ramp and a grass-and-gravel beach with a well-marked swimming area. Fishing on this 310-acre lake yields a well-mixed bag of Northern pike; cutthroat, brown, and rainbow trout; and the occasional kokanee. Wildlife viewing takes a backseat to the wealth of birds found here, but deer sightings are fairly common along the shore at dusk, and bears have been seen in the campground.

Sitting around the campfire or awakening to a symphony of birds, it's hard to imagine the bustle of activity around here during the logging-boom years of the early 1900s. Back then, this river was a super-highway used to float logs to the Blackfoot River and on to Bonner. These log drives consisted of damming up sections of the Clearwater to collect a large raft of felled logs. This wasn't a simple Huck Finn and Tom Sawyer raft; it was a serious number of trees. As a log reservoir would fill up, dynamite was used to blow the dam, allowing the load to rush into the next dammed section, where the process would be repeated until it reached Salmon Lake.

A logjam on the river could stretch for 2 miles. To prevent jams, agile men called "river hogs" or "river pigs" skillfully stepped from log to floating log, prodding them along to keep

KEY INFORMATION

ADDRESS: MT 83, Seeley Lake, MT 59868

CONTACT: 406-677-2233,
www.fs.usda.gov/lolo

OPERATED BY: Lolo National Forest

OPEN: Memorial Day weekend–Labor Day

SITES: 39 tent sites, 2 group sites

EACH SITE: Picnic table, fire grate

ASSIGNMENT: First come, first served;
no reservations for tent sites

REGISTRATION: On-site self-registration;
sites 42 and 43 are group sites that must
be reserved by calling 877-444-6777 or
visiting recreation.gov.

FACILITIES: Water spigots, vault toilets,
boat ramp, beach

PARKING: At campsites

FEE: $10, $5/extra vehicle

ELEVATION: 4,100'

RESTRICTIONS:

Pets: On leash only

Fires: In fire grates only

Alcohol: Permitted

Vehicles: 45- to 64-foot length limit;
Lake Alva is a "no wake" lake

Other: 16-day stay limit; bear-country food-
storage requirements; campground host

things moving. If a jam occurred it was their job to find the log or series of logs holding up progress and set a charge to blow them free.

Today the only objects floating on the river, besides ducks, are canoes. The Clearwater Canoe Trail is nearby and well worth your time. If you don't have a canoe, rentals are available in Seeley Lake. The trail's put-in is 8 miles south of the campground, and is clearly marked on MT 83. Allow about 2½ hours for this leisurely float. If you leave early enough, you may be able to catch a moose looking for a meal. Don't worry about a shuttle vehicle; the takeout is located at the Seeley Lake Ranger Station, which also serves as the trailhead for the level, 1.5-mile trail leading back to the parking lot.

Along the canoe trail, it's bird city. Shorebirds such as American bittern, great blue heron, and belted kingfisher will keep you entertained along the water's edge. Look a little

The Mission Mountains create a wild backdrop to Lake Alva.

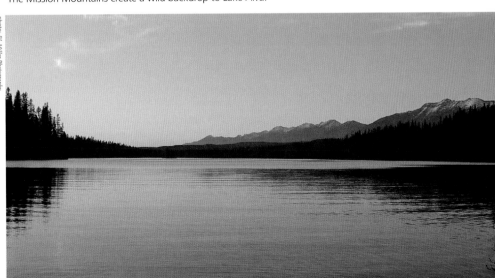

photo: RL Miller Photography

farther inland to see warblers, eagles, and osprey. When you paddle the short distance across Seeley Lake, your chances of seeing waterfowl, particularly loons, are pretty good.

If you'd rather travel by car, the Clearwater Chain-of-Lakes driving tour runs about 18 miles from Salmon Lake to Rainy Lake and provides designated viewing areas at four different lakes. It isn't quite the same as the view from the water, but you should see loons, eagles, and osprey throughout the day. (Note that the tour is closed seasonally due to bear activity in the area, so check before you go.)

Located off MT 83, 11 miles south of the campground, is Morrell Creek Road. Follow the signs to the Morrell Falls National Recreation Trail #30. This popular 5.4-mile route takes hikers through dense forests of lodgepole pine, fir, larch, and spruce on the way to Morrell Lake and Morrell Falls. It's 2.3 miles to the lake, and a view of the Swan Mountains is breathtaking. Another half mile takes you to the 90-foot double falls, where agile, fearless hikers often ascend a steep scramble to the top of the falls. Remember that this is grizzly bear country, so traveling in groups is advised.

Lake Alva Campground

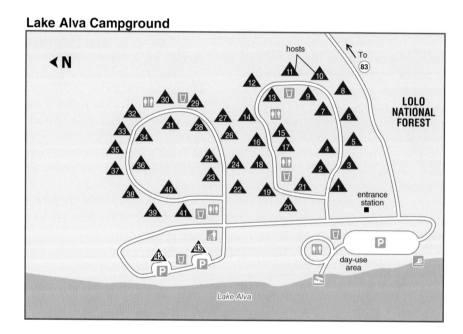

GETTING THERE

From Seeley Lake, take MT 83 north for nearly 12 miles. The campground is on the left.

GPS COORDINATES: N47° 19.393' W113° 34.991'

10

Pete Creek Campground

Beauty: ★★★★ / Privacy: ★★★★ / Quiet: ★★★★ / Spaciousness: ★★★★ / Security: ★★★★ /
Cleanliness: ★★★★★

Along the river you'll find delightful waterfalls and plenty of pools with trout and whitefish.

Three miles west of Yaak, Pete Creek is a quiet spot just off MT 508. It sits back far enough from the road that only a few sites may have bothersome road noise. Sites are well spaced, and many have a cozy, secluded feel due to the cedar, fir, larch, and spruce trees. Huge rock walls provide a dramatic backdrop and a place to challenge a budding rock climber interested in some bouldering (behind large, wooded site 8).

Sites 9–11 are three secluded and wooded walk-in sites for individuals or couples traveling light and not needing a car close by. They sit on a hilltop above Pete Creek, with a trail leading down to a nice swimming hole complete with a small beach area. Site 11 is the best of the trio, set farther off the trail and offering a little more privacy from other campers using the trail to access the creek and the Yaak River. Site 1 is small and right off the road, but it is on the creek, and a waterfall dampens the road noise. Also along the river are delightful waterfalls and plenty of pools with trout and whitefish.

Wildlife viewing is abundant, with deer, elk, and moose in the area, along with occasional sightings of mountain lions, coyotes, and grizzly and black bears. Despite the highway, this is a sparsely populated, rugged region.

Down the road, the Yaak Mercantile hums with activity. Its sparse shelves hold only the most essential items. If your tires need air, ask for the air chuck at the counter. If your whistle needs wetting, beer and pop are in the cooler. If you're planning to fish—don't fret—tackle and sage advice are readily available. You're also likely to hear what the locals think about wilderness and winter. But the Mercantile and adjoining bar are not the only game in town. Across the street, the Dirty Shame Saloon offers refreshments alongside a tiny coin laundry.

From Yaak, take South Fork Pipe Creek Road (Forest Road 68) to Vinal Lake Road (FR 746) and go north 6 miles. Here you'll find the trailhead for Vinal–Mount Henry–Boulder National Recreation Trail #9, which leads to the Mount Henry Lookout. This 16-mile round-trip requires an early start. You'll pass Turner Creek Falls and follow the ridge to get a 360-degree view from the mountaintop. Along the way, you'll see red cedars over 25 feet in diameter, probably some deer, and maybe even elk.

Another option, even though it's a 22-mile drive, is the Northwest Peaks

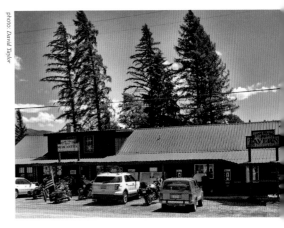

photo David Taylor

The town of Yaak is about as down-homey as you can get.

KEY INFORMATION

ADDRESS: MT 508, Yaak, MT 59935

CONTACT: 406-295-4693, www.fs.usda.gov /kootenai

OPERATED BY: Kootenai National Forest

OPEN: Year-round; full services Memorial Day weekend–Labor Day

SITES: 12

EACH SITE: Picnic table, fire grate

ASSIGNMENT: First come, first served; no reservations

REGISTRATION: On-site self-registration

FACILITIES: Water spigots, vault toilets

PARKING: At campsites

FEE: $7

ELEVATION: 2,966'

RESTRICTIONS:

Pets: On leash only

Fires: In fire rings only

Alcohol: Permitted

Vehicles: 32-foot length limit

Other: 16-day stay limit; bear-country food storage restrictions

Scenic Area. Take Pete Creek Road (FR 338) north to the trailhead, and you'll find yourself only a few miles from the Canadian and Idaho borders. There are several trails in the area, but Northwest Peak Trail #169 is an excellent day hike. This is a 4.6-mile out-and-back hike to the top of Northwest Peak (7,705'), the highest point in the Purcell Range, where you'll enjoy views of the Cabinet Mountains and Canadian Rockies in the distance. It's an easy hike, except for the final climb to the top, where the grade increases to 35 percent.

If the campground at Pete Creek is full, try Whitetail, another U.S. Forest Service site, 4 miles west on MT 508. The sites along the water here are more like an incredibly spacious backyard than a standard campground. It's a perfect place for kids to let off steam and for everyone to wade, skip rocks, and fish along this scenic stretch of the Yaak River, but it isn't as quiet as Pete Creek.

About 500 yards west of the Whitetail entrance is an open meadow where the river bends and pools, and where the original authors stumbled upon one of those rare, breathtaking moments that are easy to miss. A family of moose was calmly dining on lush aquatic vegetation. Water sparkled in the twilight as it cascaded from the bull's massive rack each time he dramatically surfaced after feasting on river-bottom delicacies. The cow and her calf frolicked downstream a hundred yards, while the Soderbergs stood mesmerized by this unexpected gift from Mother Nature after a long, hot day on the road.

Pete Creek Campground

KOOTENAI NATIONAL FOREST

GETTING THERE

From Yaak, take MT 508 southwest for 3 miles to the campground.

From Troy, take US 2 west for 10 miles to MT 508. Turn right and drive 36 miles northeast to the campground.

GPS COORDINATES: N48° 49.850' W115° 45.996'

11

△ Peters Creek Campground

Beauty: ★★★★ / Privacy: ★★★★★ / Quiet: ★★★★★ / Spaciousness: ★★★★★ / Security: ★★★ /
Cleanliness: ★★★

At this small campground, each site offers a peaceful view of the mountains.

Signs at both ends of the town of Hungry Horse read THE BEST DAM TOWN IN THE WEST, and you will certainly find some friendly people here. The town is named after—of all things—a couple of hungry horses. It's true. Tex and Jerry were hungry after wandering off during a tough winter in 1900. They both survived, and the town was named in their honor. Weird, eh?

Hungry Horse Dam, built across the South Fork of the Flathead River in 1953, is just 15 miles from the west entrance to Glacier National Park, but it doesn't get as much use as you might think. Many visitors just rush right by, not even knowing it's here.

Tucked in a narrow canyon adjacent to both the Great Bear and Bob Marshall Wilderness areas, this 34-mile-long, 3-mile-wide reservoir is up to 500 feet deep in sections and holds more than 3.5 million acre-feet of water managed both for flood control and power production. Before the reservoir was created, the native bull trout and Westslope cutthroat migrated from Flathead Lake up the Flathead River to spawn in the river's South, Middle, and North Fork tributaries. The dam's construction blocked the fish from making the annual trip to Flathead Lake, and they adapted by spawning between the South Fork of the Flathead and the Hungry Horse Reservoir. As a result, there is an unusual fishery here that is made up primarily of native species instead of introduced species like brook, brown, and rainbow trout. Visitors are requested to assist in protecting this resource by taking the time to familiarize themselves with how to identify bull trout and reviewing the most recent regulations. Fishing pressure is typically light on the reservoir, and you should find a variety of quiet spots to try your luck.

The road around Hungry Horse Reservoir is 115 miles long, and only the first 15 miles on the west side (Forest Road 895) are paved. Although the gravel surface isn't as bad as the road to Kintla Lake, it does have a reputation for eating tires. The reputation is well earned, so be prepared for a flat tire should that be your luck of the day. The nearest help is 13 bumpy miles away.

Located on the east shore (FR 38 out of Martin City), Peters Creek offers the reservoir's best option for tent camping, with sites nestled among a heavy forest of

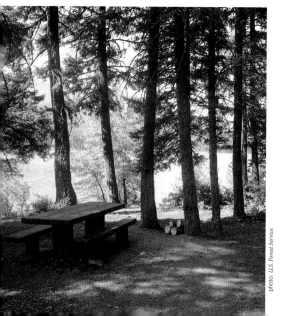

A lovely spot for a picnic

photo: *U.S. Forest Service*

KEY INFORMATION

ADDRESS: East Side Reservoir Road (Forest Road 38), Hungry Horse, MT 59919

CONTACT: 406-387-3800, www.fs.usda.gov /flathead

OPERATED BY: Flathead National Forest, Spotted Bear Ranger District

OPEN: May 15–November 30

SITES: 6

EACH SITE: Picnic table, fire grate, bear-resistant boxes at select sites

ASSIGNMENT: First come, first served; no reservations

REGISTRATION: Not required

FACILITIES: Vault toilets but no water

PARKING: At campsites

FEE: Free

ELEVATION: 3,600'

RESTRICTIONS:

Pets: On leash only

Fires: In fire rings only

Alcohol: Permitted

Vehicles: 30-foot length limit

Other: 16-day stay limit; bear-country food-storage requirements; pack in, pack out

aspens, larch, ponderosa pine, and Douglas-fir. Sites are well spaced, and each has a peaceful view of the mountains surrounding the reservoir. This is a small campground, and every site could easily be considered the best. Short trails lie behind the campsites and lead down to the reservoir and a nice area where you can enjoy a morning cup of coffee or a relaxing dinner. There is no water available at the campground itself, and the closest option is 14 miles south at Spotted Bear Campground, so be sure to bring your own.

The west-shore campgrounds (FR 895 out of Hungry Horse) pale in comparison to those on the east shore. The U.S. Forest Service has completed an assessment of the recreational facilities around the reservoir in the hope that additional funding will be made available for much-needed improvements. Many of the campgrounds are old and worn and need an infusion of TLC.

If you can't find a spot at Peters Creek, try Murray Bay (15 miles north), where some of the 18 sites have nice views of the reservoir. Another 17 miles north is Emery Bay, where seclusion is minimal but maintenance is good.

Hiking opportunities are plentiful here. The trailhead for Logan Creek Trail #62 is a few miles north on FR 38. This 12-mile round-trip enters Great Bear Wilderness area and rises more than 2,000 feet through dense forests, rugged cliffs, and wildflower meadows. Panoramic views of a lofty waterfall and Unawah and Red Top Mountains reward those who try this trail.

As you drive south on FR 38, you'll find several trailheads. At the ranger station you can continue south to Meadow Creek Gorge, where a suspension bridge crosses the designated Wild and Scenic South Fork of the Flathead River, or you can head east on FR 568 to another assortment of trailheads. Many trails in this region follow small tributaries to their headwaters in nearby alpine lakes. Be sure to get trail maps and current information from the ranger station. You'll be hiking in the wilderness, whether it's inside the official boundaries or not, and precautions and common sense are required. Problems you could encounter are far worse and more dangerous than a flat tire.

Peters Creek Campground

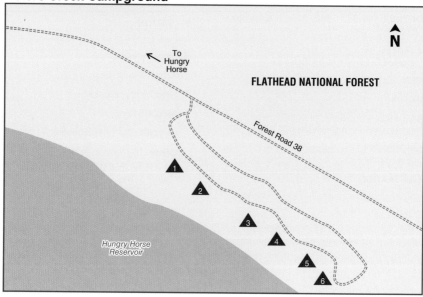

GETTING THERE

From Hungry Horse, take US 2 east for 0.6 mile. Just past the EAST SIDE HUNGRY HORSE RESERVOIR sign, turn right and go south on FR 38 for 42 miles to the campground.

GPS COORDINATES: N48° 3.487' W113° 38.744'

12

Sprague Creek Campground

Beauty: ★★★★★ / Privacy: ★★★★ / Quiet: ★★★★ / Spaciousness: ★★★★ / Security: ★★★★★ /
Cleanliness: ★★★★★

Towering cedars define this small loop on Lake McDonald.

Going-to-the-Sun Road is the only road that traverses Glacier National Park from east to west, and it is an engineering miracle. This narrow, winding road evolved between 1911 and 1933, coming in only $1 million over its original $1.5 million cost estimate (constructing it today would cost well over $90 million). For those who choose not to hike throughout the park, it provides unique access to many of the park's geologic and visual wonders. Taken from the Blackfeet name for a mountain near Logan Pass, Going-to-the-Sun Road's identity was the idea of Montana Congressman Louis C. Cramton. Fortunately, the name was shortened from "The-Face-of-Sour-Spirit-Who-Went-Back-to-the-Sun-After-His-Work-Was-Done."

During most of the year, the road appears to be going more toward the North Pole, as heavy snows create drifts up to 80 feet deep, so the opening date fluctuates from mid-May to mid-June, depending on when work crews finally get everything plowed.

Until the roadway was completed, visitors traveled through the park by foot or on horseback, spending days and weeks exploring. Today, a majority of those who enter the park spend a few hours driving Going-to-the-Sun Road and proudly proclaim they've "seen Glacier." Sadly, what they miss is an opportunity to experience this jewel by camping, hiking, or just relaxing along a creek or in a meadow to enjoy the sights, the smells, and the sounds.

Of the five campgrounds along the road, this is the best one for tenters due to its size and the restrictions against towed units. Towering cedars define this small loop on Lake McDonald, and sites range from spectacular to those that are too close for comfort. Understory is quite sparse, but most sites provide at

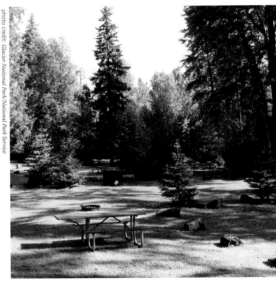

photo credit: Glacier National Park/National Park Service

Sprague Creek is one of the more relaxing campgrounds in Glacier National Park.

least some privacy. Two of the 25 sites are reserved for hikers and bicyclists and provide secure bearproof food storage, while site 8 is the most coveted for its size and incredible lake and mountain views from the picnic table. Decent lake views are also available from sites 10, 12, and 13, but there are more trees through which to peer.

Avoid sites on the inside of the loop. These sites sit on top of one another and adjoin the restrooms. They may, however, be preferable for a group of families with small children. If

KEY INFORMATION

ADDRESS: Going-to-the-Sun Road, West Glacier, MT 59936

CONTACT: 406-888-7800, nps.gov/glac

OPERATED BY: Glacier National Park

OPEN: Mid-May–mid-September

SITES: 24

EACH SITE: Picnic table, fire grate

ASSIGNMENT: First come, first served; no reservations

REGISTRATION: On-site self-registration

FACILITIES: Water spigots, flush toilets

PARKING: At campsites

FEE: $20

ELEVATION: 3,200'

RESTRICTIONS:

Pets: On leash only, not permitted on trails or along lakeshore

Fires: In fire rings only

Alcohol: Permitted

Vehicles: No towed units, only Class C RVs allowed

Other: 14-day stay limit July–Labor Day and 30-day limit the rest of the year; bear-country food storage restrictions; no firearms; no firewood gathering; special fishing regulations. No boating in Glacier at press time; call/check online for the latest information.

these or sites 20–24 are all that's left, you might want to try Fish Creek. It's not that sites 20–24 are bad, but they lack privacy and get a lot of noise from traffic on Going-to-the-Sun Road. Keep in mind that this campground fills early, and during July and August there may be days when no sites open up at all. Fish Creek is a good alternative, since it fills later in the day.

Along the lakefront is a pleasant pebbled beach with a designated swimming area. The crystalline water is fairly cold throughout the year, so wading is generally the preferred method of experiencing the lake. For those who want to fish, no license is required, and sunrise and sunset, when the wind is calm, are the best times to catch cutthroat, rainbow, and lake trout.

Within walking distance is Lake McDonald Lodge, where you can board a historic boat for tours of the lake or attend nightly programs that divulge the park's history and secrets. (*Note:* At press time in 2017, boating was prohibited in Glacier due to detection of invasive mussel, so call or check online for the latest information.) Across the road from the lodge is a trailhead leading to Fish Lake, Lincoln Lake, Mount Brown Lookout, and Sperry Chalet. The hike to Fish Lake is a 4.8-mile round-trip along Snyder Creek that gently climbs through fir and pine forests and along benches to the lake. The setting is peaceful and highlighted by the call of loons, but the heavy forest surroundings do prevent views of the mountains. Hiking to Mount Brown Lookout is a challenge. Most of this 10.8-mile trek consists of switchbacks, but there are huckleberries along the way, and the views of Lake McDonald and the surrounding mountains, including the Little Matterhorn, are awesome.

Wildlife viewing at Sprague Creek is not as good as at some of the other campgrounds due to the road traffic, but deer and elk are usually sighted in the early evening, and as dusk settles, you may hear brakes squealing as animal–vehicle collisions are avoided.

Sprague Creek Campground

GETTING THERE

From the West Glacier entrance to Glacier National Park, take Going-to-the-Sun Road northeast for 9.5 miles to the campground.

GPS COORDINATES: N48° 36.372' W113° 53.093'

13

⛺ Thompson Falls State Park Campground

Beauty: ★★★ / Privacy: ★★★★ / Quiet: ★★★★★ / Spaciousness: ★★★★★ / Security: ★★★★★ / Cleanliness: ★★★★

Easy fishing access to the world-class Clark Fork River is a prime draw.

This park is one of many places bearing the name of David Thompson, a tribute to the impact of the Canadian explorer and mapmaker. During his 28-year, 55,000-mile exploration of the Northwest, he settled nearby, from 1809 to 1811, and established a trading post, Saleesh House, named for the local Indians. The tribes demonstrated their respect for him and their awe of his telescope and mapping instruments by calling him *Koo-koo-sint* ("man who looks at the stars").

Like many campgrounds set amid a canopy of towering pines, the lack of understory affects privacy, but these sites are roomy, well spaced, and peaceful. Site 10 is unique and well designed for tenters: the tent area is perched on a terraced area set below the picnic table and fire ring, which mitigates the open view to site 11 across the road. The most popular site is 7 because it overlooks the Clark Fork River, but it is next to the boat ramp and its daytime bustle. River access is also easy from sites 15, 16, and 17. They aren't exactly riverfront but do adjoin a short trail to the Clark Fork.

Even though a group site occupies its own corner close to the access road and large RVs do camp here, the campground host keeps everyone under control and maintains quiet. As a result, deer are usually spotted several times a day by kids riding their bikes around the campground loops. Osprey sightings are frequent as well.

The nearby Clark Fork River is an obvious draw for anglers camping at Thompson Falls State Park.

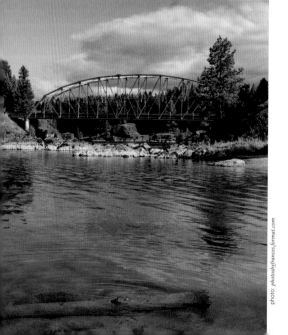

Fishing in the Clark Fork is a prime draw, particularly for fly-fishing devotees. But this world-class river is tricky, and novices may want to focus on the experience rather than the quantity of their catch. Rainbow, brown, and cutthroat trout, along with largemouth and smallmouth bass, are prevalent, and rods and reels are available in town for those who aren't equipped but can't resist the temptation to wet a line.

Floating the Clark Fork is an excellent way to spend a sunny day, whether you're in a raft or canoe. Inner tubes are often the craft of choice for the young (and the young at heart), and since the river runs along the highway, shuttles are fairly easy. If you are planning a long float, outfitters and supplies are available in Thompson Falls.

photo: *photosbyfrances.format.com*

KEY INFORMATION

ADDRESS: 2220 Blue Slide Road, Thompson Falls, MT 59873

CONTACT: 406-751-4590, stateparks.mt.gov /thompson-falls; reservations: reserve america.com

OPERATED BY: Thompson Falls State Park

OPEN: May–September

SITES: 16, plus 1 group site

EACH SITE: Picnic table; fire grate

ASSIGNMENT: First come, first served or by reservation

REGISTRATION: At office or on-site self-registration

FACILITIES: Water spigots, vault toilets, boat ramp, picnic shelters

PARKING: At campsites

FEE: $18 resident, $28 nonresident; $6/extra nonresident vehicle

ELEVATION: 2,362′

RESTRICTIONS:

Pets: On leash only

Fires: In fire rings only

Alcohol: Permitted

Vehicles: 35-foot length limit

Other: 16-day stay limit; bear-country food-storage requirements

When you're ready to explore the area, don't spend your time looking for the falls in the park's name; they disappeared years ago when the Clark Fork was dammed, but a variety of other sights are nearby. In town, a pedestrian bridge leads to a river island with several nature trails—prime territory for wildlife enthusiasts. Three miles southeast on MT 200 is the Mount Silcox Wildlife Management Area, where white-tailed and mule deer, elk, black bears, and turkey are visible throughout the summer, and mountain goats can be seen on the surrounding cliffs. KooKooSint Sheep Viewing Area is another 5 miles south on MT 200. Although peak viewing opportunities are during the fall mating season, sightings are still possible during the summer, when sheep perch on the rocky outcrops.

The state's best huckleberry-hunting country is found throughout this area. You can try asking locals for suggestions, but most patches are closely guarded secrets. Don't be afraid to strike out on your own beginning about mid-June at lower elevations and into July for the higher mountainsides. Patches sprout at elevations between 3,500 and 7,000 feet, where tree cover is less than 50 percent and they can receive necessary sunlight. Burn areas that are a few decades old are also good possibilities for patches, as are south-facing slopes. Generally, no permit is required to pick up to 10 gallons per person, but check with the U.S. Forest Service on current regulations, and be sure your newfound berry patch isn't on private land before you pick.

A drive along the Vermilion River on Blue Slide Road (off MT 200 at the Trout Creek Bridge) brings you to a short hike down to the waterfall and a great picnic spot. Trailheads for several longer trails dot both sides of this forest road, and most follow a creek or stream.

West of Thompson Falls on Prospect Creek Road is Blossom Lake Trail #404. You may share the way with an occasional horseback party, but it isn't a problem on this isolated, 10-mile round-trip to a series of high mountain lakes. The trail itself runs along the Idaho–Montana border, and your trek can continue all the way to the Coeur d'Alene River near Lookout Pass.

Thompson Falls State Park Campground

GETTING THERE

From Thompson Falls, take MT 200 northwest for 1 mile (milepost 50). Turn right into the campground.

GPS COORDINATES: N47° 36.975' W115° 23.206'

NORTH CENTRAL MONTANA

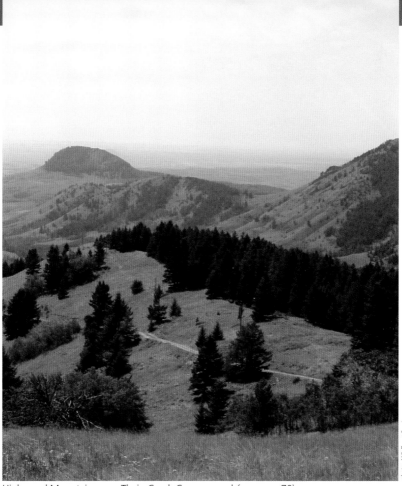

Highwood Mountains near Thain Creek Campground *(see page 70)*

photo: *U.S. Forest Service*

14

Cave Mountain Campground

Beauty: ★★★★★ / Privacy: ★★★★★ / Quiet: ★★★★★ / Spaciousness: ★★★★★ / Security: ★★★ /
Cleanliness: ★★★★★

Enjoy spectacular vistas of the Rocky Mountains as you drive along the Teton River.

Views of the Rocky Mountain front are spectacular as you drive along the Teton River to Cave Mountain. Ahead of you are Wind Mountain and flat-topped Ear Mountain. This is actually part of the original Old North Trail, used for centuries as a travel corridor between Canada and points south. Limestone cliffs rise 500 feet on either side of you, and viewpoints provide panoramic 360-degree vistas.

The road enters a gap in the cliffs, and not far beyond, a sign points the way to Cave Mountain. Two bridge crossings, one over the North Fork Teton River and one over the Middle Fork, lead to the campground entrance. Set under a beautiful mix of birch, aspen, and pine, the campground's 18 sites are perfect for tenters looking for quiet and solitude. Sites here are spacious, and sites 1, 3, 4, 6, 8, 10, and 12 back up to and are only a short walk from the North Fork of the Teton. You won't go wrong picking any one of these pine needle–covered sites. Site 14, on the back end of the loop at the end of the road, is nicely secluded. Sites 5 and 7 are also well separated, with plenty of space to spread out for a few days.

photo: Steve Pattisas

Hikers make their way to Mount Wright.

This campground makes a great base camp for fishing, hiking, or mountain biking. The trailhead for Middle Fork Teton River Trail #108 is at Cave Mountain. It's actually more of a stroll than a hike, as it follows the river bottoms: no mountain vistas, no dramatic canyons, just a walk in the woods along a stream where you can relax, watch industrious beavers, or fish for mountain whitefish or trout. From this trail you can also access the Bob Marshall Wilderness.

A mile east of the campground is the trailhead for Clary Coulee Trail #177. This 12-mile out-and-back trail follows an open bench with views of vast plains to the east and Rocky Mountain peaks to the west. Small stream crossings necessitate some short, steep up-and-down climbs, but overall this is a moderate trail that isn't heavily used.

Another hiking option is North Fork Teton Trail #107, which winds along the river through narrow Box Canyon. During summer, the many river crossings on this trail are pretty simple, but during spring runoff, it's quite possible that the depth and speed of the

KEY INFORMATION

ADDRESS: Canyon Road (County Road 144), Choteau, MT 59422

CONTACT: 406-466-5341, www.fs.usda.gov/helena

OPERATED BY: Helena–Lewis and Clark National Forest, Rocky Mountain Ranger District

OPEN: Memorial Day weekend–October

SITES: 18

EACH SITE: Picnic table, fire grate

ASSIGNMENT: First come, first served; no reservations

REGISTRATION: On-site self-registration

FACILITIES: Hand-pump well, vault toilets

PARKING: At campsites

FEE: $6

ELEVATION: 5,200'

RESTRICTIONS:

Pets: On leash only

Fires: In fire rings only

Alcohol: Permitted

Vehicles: 35-foot length limit

Other: 16-day stay limit; pack in, pack out; bear-country food storage restrictions

---

water will make them impassable. The trailhead for this 8-mile out-and-back trip is 4 miles west of the campground.

You can climb to the peak of Mount Wright on a day hike from the trailhead 10 miles west of the campground. The trail follows West Fork Trail #144 for the first quarter mile, and from there it's a steep 4-mile climb through prime habitat for mountain goats and bighorn sheep. The descent can be challenging as well, but if you're in good shape, the view from the 8,875-foot summit is spectacular and worth the effort. On a clear day you'll see peaks at Glacier National Park and part of the Chinese Wall running through the Bob Marshall Wilderness.

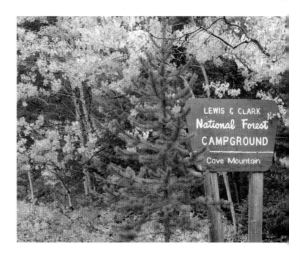

About 5 miles east of the campground is a turnoff for Our Lake Trail and the Pine Butte Preserve, a 15,000-acre wetland owned by The Nature Conservancy that provides significant grizzly bear habitat. In order to preserve undisturbed habitat for the grizzlies, the 0.25-mile A. B. Guthrie Memorial Trail is the only hiking access provided. The 300-foot elevation gain allows views of a portion of the fen wetland complex and

A formal welcome to Cave Mountain Campground

of limber pine savanna. You may not see any bears while you're here, but dozens of other mammals like elk, deer, and coyote may draw your attention. More than 100 bird species have been sighted here, from songbirds to sandhill cranes.

If you're heading for the trails instead of the preserve, take a right after you cross the river and follow South Fork Road (Forest Road 109) for 9 miles to the trailhead. Our Lake

Trail #184 is a 5-mile out-and-back that climbs steeply in places and can be slippery before the snow melts in late June. Bears are seen often in this area, and many people see mountain goats clinging to the slopes on the other side of the lake. A waterfall about halfway to the lake is usually less crowded than the lake itself. If you are thinking about making this an overnight hike, camping is allowed near the waterfall, but not near the lake.

The Choteau area is famous for more than ranching and spectacular scenery. Nearby Egg Mountain is where paleontologist Jack Horner discovered fossilized dinosaur eggs and embryos, establishing the Willow Creek Anticline as an active site where finds are still being made. If you want to take part in a dig, stop at the Two Medicine Dinosaur Center in Bynum for information.

Cave Mountain Campground

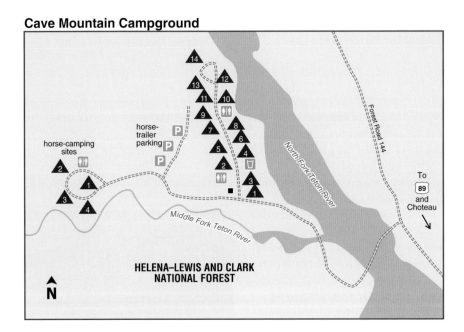

GETTING THERE

From Choteau, take US 89 north for 4 miles to the TETON PASS WINTER SPORTS AREA and EUREKA RESERVOIR signs. Turn left at the signs, onto FR 144, and go 23 miles to the campground. The last 5 miles are gravel and dirt.

GPS COORDINATES: N47° 53.483' W112° 43.617'

15

Home Gulch Campground

Beauty: ★★★★★ / Privacy: ★★★★ / Quiet: ★★★★ / Spaciousness: ★★★ / Security: ★★★★ / Cleanliness: ★★★★

This spectacular canyon invites tenters to make camp in the shadow of overthrust formations along the shoreline.

The Sun River glistens in this steep canyon as it flows east from its headwaters in the Bob Marshall Wilderness. Only a shadow of its former wild self, the Sun is now tamed by the Gibson Dam. The landscape is dramatic here where plains collide with the leading edge of the Rocky Mountain front. Combine the setting with the wealth of wildlife, and it's easy to understand the river's importance to the Blackfeet Indians. To them this is Medicine River, a part of their homeland that valiant ancestors fought to protect. It was included within the original Blackfeet Reservation boundaries in 1855, but as the boundaries were redefined in 1865, 1868, and 1873, the tribe's territory shrank. Today the reservation boundaries are over 50 miles away.

As you drive to the campground along Sun Canyon Road you'll see a bighorn-sheep viewing area. One of the largest herds in North America lives here, lured by the same spectacular topography that invites tenters to make camp in the shadow of overthrust formations along the shoreline. Set among thick stands of aspens, the sites are well spaced, and most have a nice amount of ground cover providing privacy between them. Eight sites have river access, with paths leading to fishing, wading, or stone skipping in the cold, clear water. Water levels in the river can fluctuate significantly depending on discharge from the reservoir, but fishing is still good for rainbow, brown, and cutthroat trout in the deep pools throughout the canyon.

Rafting the Sun River's 3 miles of Class V whitewater just west of Home Gulch can be a challenge even for experienced rafters. Fishing from boats is not allowed here for obvious reasons. The section through the canyon and Home Gulch is a little calmer, with Class II and III rapids, but rocks and underwater ledges are frequent in this section. Beyond the canyon to Willow Creek Reservoir, the river winds and twists relentlessly, with some occasional Class II spots.

To the east is Sun River Wildlife Management Area, winter home to one of the state's largest elk populations. The WMA's 20,000 acres are open to the public in summer, and visitors can hike, bike, or drive throughout the area to see wetlands, wildlife, and maybe a black or grizzly bear set against a magnificent backdrop.

Mortimer Gulch Campground lies 2.5 miles west. This camping alternative sits directly on the reservoir and is a major trailhead, but it's usually full of

The gorgeous and glistening Sun River

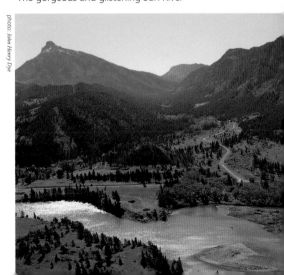

photo: John Henry Dye

RVs and motorboats. If you do decide to camp here, you'll choose between two loops. Sites 18–20, on the first loop you'll encounter, are large and more secluded than the others. You won't be right on the water at any of the sites here, but you'll be close enough to still hear an occasional boat motor during the day.

Home Gulch–Lime Trail #267 is a 15-mile point-to-point hike with gentle grade changes. The scenery is spectacular, but don't forget to turn back before you're exhausted. Not heavily used, this trail is ideal for families or those looking for easy terrain. The trailhead is 0.5 miles from Home Gulch, north of the Sun Canyon Lodge gate.

A variety of trails lead from the area into the Bob Marshall Wilderness to the northwest. Just past Home Gulch is Hannan Gulch Trail #240, which begins near the guard station and climbs nearly 2,400 feet along its 6.5-mile length to the head of the gulch. This is a good mountain-bike trail due to its width and relatively low usage by hikers.

Mortimer Gulch Trail #252 begins at Mortimer Gulch Campground and runs the 7-mile length of the gulch to Blacktail Creek Trail #223. It's surprising that this isn't a more heavily used trail, since the elevation gain is minimal and it provides excellent views of Sawtooth Ridge, Norwegian and French Gulches, and Gibson Reservoir. This is an especially good wildlife-viewing area in the spring and early summer before the deer, elk, mountain goats, and bighorn sheep head for higher elevations.

Campsite at Home Gulch

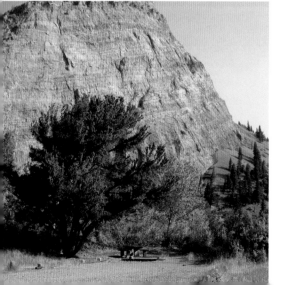

North Fork Sun River Trail #201 also begins at the Mortimer trailhead. This trail follows the north side of Gibson Reservoir for 2 miles before it intersects with Big George Gulch Trail #251, a more difficult trail that continues another 6 miles on a high bench. The trail drops and climbs steeply in sections over the pass, but switchbacks ease the effort. Views to the south are of Sawtooth Ridge and Gibson Reservoir, and you'll see plenty of wildlife here as well.

Home Gulch Campground

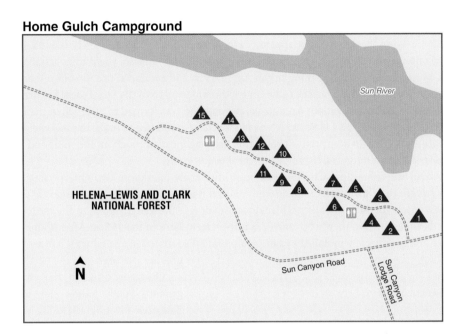

GETTING THERE

From Augusta, take Manix Street west toward Gibson Reservoir for 3.7 miles; this road turns into Forest Road 108. At the intersection with the sign for the reservoir, turn right and go 16.8 miles on Sun Canyon Road (FR 180). Turn right at the sign to the campground.

GPS COORDINATES: N47° 36.950' W112° 43.467'

16

Kading Campground

Beauty: ★★★ / Privacy: ★★★★ / Quiet: ★★★★ / Spaciousness: ★★★★★ / Security: ★★★★ / Cleanliness: ★★★★★

Brook trout are easy to catch in the pools of cool water held back by downed logs and large rocks.

While the Little Blackfoot Valley appears virtually unpopulated, it has been home to a variety of enterprises. Shortly after you turn onto Little Blackfoot Road, you'll come to Charter Oak Mine. This abandoned mine began life in 1916 and produced ore for more than 40 years. In the 1990s, the complex came under the supervision of the U.S. Forest Service for reclamation and preservation. An unusual partnership was formed in 2001 when the Helena National Forest and a class at Helena High School combined to make improvements at the site and create an interpretive trail. Numbered signposts throughout the mine and mill correspond to an interpretive brochure available at the site.

About the same time Charter Oak began full-scale operation, two enterprising settlers sought their fortune from a different natural resource. You'll see the remains of their handiwork if you take the hike to Blackfoot Meadows. The marshy pond in the meadows was dammed by two men who started a beaver farm here in the 1920s. After about five years, the economic windfall they anticipated failed to materialize, and they left seeking greener pastures.

The Little Blackfoot River hosts a splendid brook trout fishery.

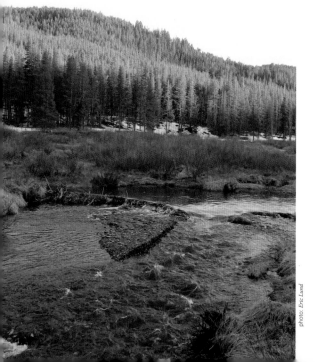

photo: Eric Lund

On your drive to the campground, you'll follow the Little Blackfoot River almost to its headwaters. Along the way, watch for white-tailed deer and small mammals in the roadside meadows, and those who are especially observant should see raptors or grouse.

Nestled on the west side of the Continental Divide along a trout-filled river, Kading is a popular weekend escape for those in Helena and the surrounding communities. On weekdays, however, you will likely have your choice of sites to set up camp. Sites here are spacious, but unfortunately the campground is part of an area affected by a pine beetle infestation in recent years, necessitating tree removal, so seclusion and beauty have taken something of a hit.

KEY INFORMATION

ADDRESS: Little Blackfoot Road
(Forest Road 227), Elliston, MT 59728

CONTACT: 406-449-5201,
www.fs.usda.gov/helena

OPERATED BY: Helena–Lewis and Clark
National Forest, Helena Ranger District

OPEN: June–September

SITES: 11

EACH SITE: Picnic table, fire grate

ASSIGNMENT: First come, first served;
no reservations

REGISTRATION: On-site self-registration

FACILITIES: Hand-pump water, vault toilets

PARKING: At campsites

FEE: $8

ELEVATION: 6,200'

RESTRICTIONS:

Pets: On leash only

Fires: In fire rings only

Alcohol: Permitted

Vehicles: 30-foot length limit

Other: 16-day stay limit; bear-country
food storage restrictions; pack in,
pack out

Sites 1, 2, 4, and 5, on the river side of the road, lie closest to the riverbank, which makes dropping a line or casting a fly extremely easy. The downside is their proximity to the day-use parking areas. Sites 8 and 10, on the river side at the end of the road, are quieter but farther from the water.

The Little Blackfoot is narrow here, and brook trout are plentiful. They're easy to catch in the pools of cool water held back by downed logs and large rocks, making this a great stop for those with young anglers in tow. Not as plentiful, but very much in evidence, are rainbow and brown trout along with longnose suckers. Bull trout are also found here, so be sure you're current on fishing regulations.

Choose from a variety of hiking opportunities. You can easily spend a few days here exploring the area. For starters, try the easy 11-mile out-and-back hike to Blackfoot Meadow Trail #329, which begins from the trailhead half a mile past the campground. The trail runs for about a mile along an old road until you take the fork that gently heads down to the riverbank and across a small bridge. The next section is fairly marshy, so keep that in mind when you're selecting footgear. The surrounding hillsides are painted in beargrass, Indian paintbrush, bluebells, and grouse whortleberry (where, you guessed it, grouse like to hang out). There is nothing as heart-stopping on a leisurely hike as a grouse bursting into flight only a few feet away from you! There will be another river crossing where you can try the downed logs or just wade across. Another mile or so brings you mountain views and the broad, wildflower-strewn Blackfoot Meadow. Relax and have lunch here before retracing your route to the campground.

Both mountain bikers and hikers may want to take a 13-mile loop that follows Trail #329 to Blackfoot Meadow and then continues northeast on Trail #362 to the ridge, picking up Trail #359. This trail takes you into Larabee Gulch and ends at Forest Road 227. From there it's 2 miles west to the campground to complete the loop.

Adjacent to the campground is Kading Cabin, named for the area rancher who originally owned the land and built by the Civilian Conservation Corps in the 1930s. Today it is a year-round rental cabin and the site of various Forest Service summer programs.

Kading Campground

GETTING THERE

From Elliston, take US 12 east for 1 mile to Little Blackfoot Road (FR 227). Turn right and go 13 miles southwest to the campground.

From Helena, take US 12 west for 18.5 miles to Little Blackfoot Road (FR 227). Turn left and go 13 miles southwest to the campground.

GPS COORDINATES: N46° 25.733' W112° 28.883'

17

⚠ Logging Creek Campground

Beauty: ★★★★ / Privacy: ★★★★★ / Quiet: ★★★★★ / Spaciousness: ★★★★ / Security: ★★★ /
Cleanliness: ★★★★

Camping here is as relaxing as watching the creek flow.

The two routes into Logging Creek are as diverse as the countryside. On the tamer ride along MT 227, your teeth won't chatter nearly as much as they will on the narrow, single-lane track called Logging Creek Road. If you're in a rental car or you've borrowed a good friend's Lexus, you should seriously consider the highway route, unless you're willing to risk your insurance or your friendship.

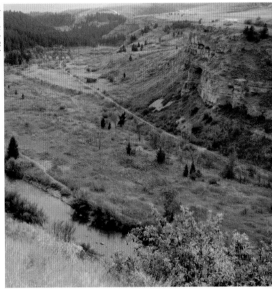

photo: Linda Blakeman

Logging Creek is tucked on the northern edge of the Little Belt Mountains. Your drive in will be a visual education about the Madison Limestone Formation that makes the views around this campground worth the drive. This formation lies beneath much of Montana's surface and is unique because of the many caves, fissures, and seams that allow water to run through it. It's like a giant slab of Swiss cheese. Water enters above the surface, but in some places it moves beneath the surface and splits off in many directions, all the while continuing to flow downhill. Surrounding this limestone formation are other geologic formations that developed before and after the limestone; these formations seal the water into the porous rock channel.

A top-down view of Belt Creek and trails adjacent to Sluice Boxes State Park

No matter which route you take, you will cross Belt Creek, which is a great example of how the Madison Limestone Formation works. At certain points, during periods of low water, the creekbed runs dry while the upstream and downstream ends continue to flow. After staying at Logging Creek, visit Giant Springs State Park in Great Falls. The pristine water flowing from these springs originated in the Little Belt Mountains that surround Logging Creek. But don't expect the water flowing underground today to come out at Giant Springs next week. It takes thousands of years for each drop of water to make the circuitous underground trip.

Belt Creek also runs through nearby Sluice Boxes State Park, a narrow box canyon sliced into the limestone. The park's name comes from the water cascading down a limestone formation that resembles a miner's sluice box. Hiking here requires several creek crossings, which often aren't possible until well into the summer. While you're hiking, imagine the complexity of moving train cars filled with limestone across these cliffs. You'll even find remnants of an old mining town awaiting exploration.

KEY INFORMATION

ADDRESS: Forest Road 839, Great Falls, MT 59401

CONTACT: 406-236-5100, www.fs.usda.gov/helena

OPERATED BY: Helena–Lewis and Clark National Forest, Belt Creek Ranger District

OPEN: Memorial Day weekend–October, weather permitting

SITES: 26

EACH SITE: Picnic table, fire grate; upright grill at some sites

ASSIGNMENT: First come, first served; no reservations

REGISTRATION: On-site self-registration

FACILITIES: Hand-pump well, vault toilets

PARKING: At campsites

FEE: $10

ELEVATION: 4,500'

RESTRICTIONS:

Pets: On leash only

Fires: In fire rings only

Alcohol: Permitted

Vehicles: 30-foot length limit

Other: 16-day stay limit; pack in, pack out; bear-country food-storage requirements

Camping at Logging Creek is as relaxing as the flowing creek itself. Well-spaced sites sit among aspen and fir trees. Undergrowth is thin, so you will see your neighbors. Any of the sites along the creek are good, but 14 and 16 are favorites for their size and access. Sites 24–26 have an extra benefit in their proximity to the best wading spot on the creek. Over the years, amateur engineers have built an impressive ring of rocks pooling the water, and children of all ages can be found cooling off here. Wildlife visits the campground on a regular basis, and at least a few bears stop by every summer. Views of the limestone cliffs are dramatic, and exploring them from the creek is a good choice. When you find a perch, relax and watch the anglers below trying to outsmart the trout.

A trailhead 3 miles south on Forest Road 839 at Mill Creek is the starting point for a variety of hikes. North Fork Deep Creek Trail #303 isn't an easy trail, but it does provide fishing access to the Smith River and its namesake creek. The 8.8-mile trail sees heavy use by hikers, motorized vehicles, and horses, and it ends at Deep Creek. After a mile on Trail #303, there is a junction with Ming-Coulee Trail #307. Several good vista points dot this trail, and you might even see a few deer.

Other trails spur off from these trails for a variety of hiking options. You'll encounter fewer motorized travelers if you visit during the week. Some of these trails cross private land or require starting from a trailhead on private land. The landowners have agreed to provide access, but you must request permission first. Information about these trails can be found on the signboards at the fee station. Mountain bikers will find any of the trail options rewarding. Taking longer day trips only involves looping onto another trail.

Logging Creek Campground

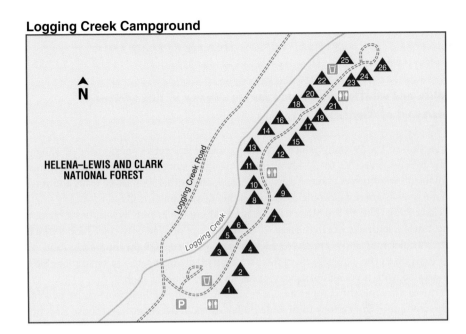

HELENA–LEWIS AND CLARK
NATIONAL FOREST

GETTING THERE

From Great Falls, take US 87/US 89 southeast 40 miles to Armington Junction. Turn right and continue 10 miles on US 89 to Evans–Riceville Road. Turn right and go 7 miles to the Y intersection. Bear left onto a single-lane dirt-and-gravel road and go 4.4 miles to the campground sign at FR 839. Turn right and drive 2.2 miles to the campground.

From Monarch, take US 89 north for 3 miles to Logging Creek Road (County Road 427). Make a sharp left turn and go 11.2 miles to a Y intersection. Bear left and drive 2.2 miles to the campground. (*Note:* This route is not recommended for low-clearance vehicles or RVs.)

GPS COORDINATES: N47° 6.067' W111° 0.533'

18

Many Pines Campground

Beauty: ★★★★ / Privacy: ★★★ / Quiet: ★★★ / Spaciousness: ★★★★ / Security: ★★★★ /
Cleanliness: ★★★★★

Wildlife and wildflowers abound during summer in this somewhat hidden part of Montana.

The section of US 89 along which this campground is located—designated at Kings Hill Scenic Byway—stretches for 71 lovely miles through a somewhat hidden part of Montana. Wildlife and wildflowers abound during summer, and with 450 miles of trails and roads to explore, crowds are not a problem except on the most popular trails.

Many Pines, like all the other campgrounds along the Scenic Byway, has a bit of road noise, but the setting is worth it. Here, 22 campsites are divided between a loop to the right of the entrance road and a straight segment along Belt Creek. On the loop, sites 6 and 7 both have steps up to the campsite from the parking pad, giving a sense of separation. Site 8 is well isolated, with no neighboring campsites on this end of the loop.

True to its name, the campground is set in a thick stand of lodgepole pines, which limits the amount of understory to provide buffer zones between sites. Of those sites on the creek-road segment, sites 15, 16, and 19 have greater privacy than their neighbors. Half of the sites overlook the creek, but they are also closer to the occasional buzz from the highway. Wading in the creek is fun on hot days, and trout fishing can be rewarding, but check regulations, as some may be strictly catch and release.

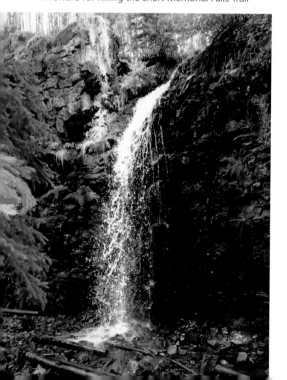

A reward for hiking the short Memorial Falls Trail

Neihart (population 51) is the only town you will find between Monarch to the north and White Sulphur Springs to the south. It's a small, friendly place where folks are ready to fill your coffee cup or pour a cold drink and discuss everything from politics to the weather. Just north of town, an area of exposed Precambrian rock enticed miners to stop and explore this mineral-rich area. The discovery of lead, silver, zinc, gold, and sapphires brought an onslaught of treasure-seekers to the heart of the Little Belt Mountains. Established in 1881, Neihart has survived the continuing boom-and-bust life cycles of a mining town. Look carefully and you'll see evidence of mining history. Can you find the old false-front building bearing the sign, WU TANG, LAUNDRY, DRUGS 1882?

Another treasure lies above ground, exposed to the impact of the elements,

KEY INFORMATION

ADDRESS: US 89, Great Falls, MT 59401

CONTACT: 406-236-5100,
www.fs.usda.gov/helena

OPERATED BY: Helena–Lewis and
Clark National Forest, Belt Creek
Ranger District

OPEN: Memorial Day weekend–
September

SITES: 22

EACH SITE: Picnic table, fire grate

ASSIGNMENT: First come, first served;
no reservations

REGISTRATION: On-site self-registration

FACILITIES: Hand-pump well, vault toilets

PARKING: At campsites

FEE: $10

ELEVATION: 5,900'

RESTRICTIONS:

Pets: On leash only

Fires: In fire ring only

Alcohol: Permitted

Vehicles: 45-foot length limit

Other: 16-day stay limit; pack in, pack out;
bear-country food storage restrictions

---

mankind, and fire. The surrounding forest, a treasure of incalculable value, is guarded by day from the Porphyry Peak fire lookout. Open to visitors, this operational fire watch is one of a shrinking core of fire towers in Montana, as new technology takes over. Fortunately, many towers are old enough to be listed as historic structures, and this may help save them from ultimately being dismantled.

The ranger in the Porphyry Peak tower watches for fire using the same methods that have been used for decades—with a few twists. The tower has a high-speed Internet connection allowing the ranger to check weather and fire data, records of area lightning strikes, and the ability to input GPS coordinates from people in the field to help pinpoint a fire start.

Not everyone is comfortable spending hours upon hours alone, perched above the treetops, watching and waiting. The rewards can be priceless, however: a bird's-eye view of the Northern Lights, the chance to watch bears from a safe vantage point, and making calls to prevent disaster.

Just north of the campground, a turnoff leads to the Memorial Falls Trail #321 for an easy 15-minute walk to two spectacular waterfalls. Other hiking options with trailheads off US 89 are nearby.

During summer flows, Belt Creek is a great place to cool off and have some fun.

Paine Gulch Trail #737 is a 7.6-mile out-and-back to Paine Gulch Creek and the base of Servoss Mountain. This easy trail begins 1 mile south of Monarch and is one of a few in the area designated as off limits to motorized vehicles. Two more difficult trails begin at the Belt Creek Ranger Station, where the staff can assist you with maps and contact information.

Access to the Tenderfoot Creek Trail System is west of Kings Hill Campground on Forest Service Road 839. The main Tenderfoot Trail #342 winds down to the creek, and many day visitors frequent this area to fish for trout. Additional trail spurs can be combined for loop hikes throughout the canyon. As with many other trails, several creek crossings may not be passable during spring runoff. Armed with a trail map, plenty of water, and sunscreen, you'll find that the potential for finding a place of solitude exists if you're persistent.

Many Pines Campground

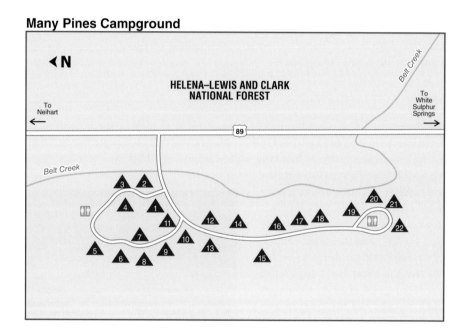

GETTING THERE

From Neihart, take US 89 south for 2.7 miles to the campground.

GPS COORDINATES: N46° 53.883' W110° 41.433'

19

Park Lake Campground

Beauty: ★★★ / Privacy: ★★★ / Quiet: ★★★ / Spaciousness: ★★★★ / Security: ★★★★★ / Cleanliness: ★★★★

The lake's clear water shimmers against lushly forested mountains.

Five-acre Park Lake appears as a thoughtful gift from Mother Nature. In reality, it is man-made, part of a late-1800s mountain reservoir system built to provide water for mining operations farther down the mountain. Unlike the mines in nearby Butte, here the treasure was silver, not copper, and the ore mined from this area was so rich that taking it to Fort Benton and shipping it to Swansea, Wales, still created a significant profit for the mining companies. Millions of dollars' worth of silver was extracted in the 1890s alone, and reminders of mining history are prevalent for those who take the time to explore.

Park Lake, with its clear blue water shimmering against the mountains, proves that not every remnant of placer mining is a blight on the landscape. Keep this setting in mind to soften the hammering you'll encounter on the access road's washboard sections on the climb into the Boulder Mountains. Always a popular escape for Helena Valley residents, this area may be a bit too noisy for those seeking a quiet weekend getaway. But come Monday, the area returns to its placid mountain splendor.

Like Kading Campground (see page 58), Park Lake lies in an area of Helena–Lewis and Clark National Forest that was struck by a pine beetle infestation several years ago, making it necessary to remove standing dead trees from the campground for visitor safety. Privacy and beauty, therefore, are not quite what they once were.

The 22 campsites set along the looped road provide the perfect place to set up base camp for a multiday stay. Large boulders provide natural play structures for a game of "king of the rock" or a place to perch while reading a book. Site 17, at the back of the loop, is somewhat removed from the other sites. A few steps down from the parking spur take you to the picnic table and fire ring, and farther below is a great space to pitch a tent. Site 15, also on the back of the loop, is large as well. These sites are farther from the lake, but since none of the sites is lakefront and it isn't that far away, the relative privacy is a nice perk. Site 10 is very large and has access to both the trail to the lake and the trail to the wetland area.

For those who venture here before mid-June, be prepared for sudden snow squalls one day and blue skies and balmy temperatures the next; temperature fluctuations of 40 degrees or more are not uncommon. Summer weather settles in

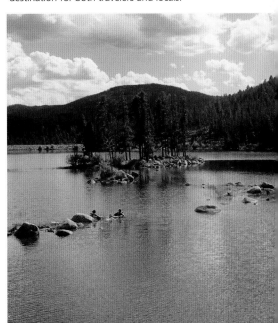

Picturesque and spacious, Park Lake is a popular destination for both travelers and locals.

KEY INFORMATION

ADDRESS: Forest Road 4009, Clancy, MT 59634

CONTACT: 406-449-5201, www.fs.usda.gov/helena

OPERATED BY: Helena–Lewis and Clark National Forest, Helena Ranger District

OPEN: May–November

SITES: 22

EACH SITE: Picnic table, fire grate

ASSIGNMENT: First come, first served; no reservations

REGISTRATION: On-site self-registration

FACILITIES: Water spigots, vault toilets, boat launch

PARKING: At campsites

FEE: $8

ELEVATION: 6,360'

RESTRICTIONS:

Pets: On leash only

Fires: In fire rings only

Alcohol: Permitted

Vehicles: 30-foot length limit

Other: 16-day stay limit; nonmotorized boats only

---

during July and August, and sites fill quickly on Fridays when the weather is good, but during the week you will find yourself with very few, if any, neighbors.

Most people spend at least part of their time here on the water—boating, swimming, or fishing. The lake supports a healthy population of Arctic grayling, rainbow trout, and Yel-

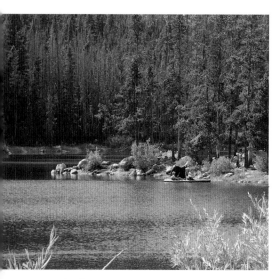

An island getaway in Park Lake

lowstone cutthroat trout, and the restriction against motors makes a canoe- or float tube–fishing excursion with fly rod in hand an enticing option. This 5-acre lake is crystal clear, and its tiny islands make good resting places for one or two people. There's no designated beach area, but many visitors wade and swim from several access points. Lakefront picnic sites are well spaced.

Nearby hiking trails offer a variety of day hikes, ranging from a 2-mile hike around the lake to short spurs leading away from the campground. As you hike around the lake you'll see remnants of mining cabins and many wildflowers. Full-day hiking routes head toward the Continental Divide and other tiny lakes, or you can take a loop around Frohner or Cataract Basin. Mountain bikers have plenty of options, although you will be sharing those nice wide trails with four-wheelers on occasion. The trailhead for Lava Mountain Trail #244 is about a mile north of Park Lake and is probably the best choice for bikers. This 8-mile trail is wide but steep and will challenge hikers and bikers alike.

At this altitude, the wealth of surrounding wetlands doesn't attract a lot of mosquitoes, but it does provide an excellent habitat for a variety of species. Hiking from the campground can be rewarded with a view of moose, elk, black bear, mule deer, and even hard-to-spot wolverines. The potential for wildlife-viewing and bird-watching, combined with excellent fishing and nearby trails, makes this site a gold mine for campers.

Park Lake Campground

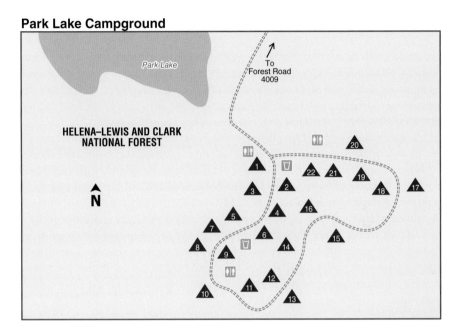

GETTING THERE

From Clancy, take Exit 182 off I-15 south of Helena. Following the signs for Park Lake, go 7.3 miles northwest on Lump Gulch Road to the Y intersection. Take Forest Road 4009 southwest for 6.2 miles to the campground.

GPS COORDINATES: N46° 26.567' W112° 10.117'

20

Thain Creek Campground

Beauty: ★★★★ / Privacy: ★★★★★ / Quiet: ★★★★ / Spaciousness: ★★★★ / Security: ★★★★ / Cleanliness: ★★★★★

Streams in the Highwood Mountains carve a colorful quilt of meadows and forests filled with wildflowers and wildlife.

The route to Thain Creek travels through ranch country in the lowlands of the Highwood Mountains. Named *Espi-toh-tok* by the Blackfeet Indians due to the timber that runs high along its slopes, this is one of Montana's dozen island mountain ranges, created by volcanic eruptions over 50 million years ago. Streams carve a colorful quilt of meadows and forests filled with wildflowers and wildlife, and ranches seem to stretch forever.

While gold miners were seeking their fortune to the west, cattlemen began staking their claims as well. Expansive ranches spread across open prairies and mountain valleys, and cattle became as commonplace as antelope. This is open rangeland, with cattle grazing throughout the national forest. Every fall, cowboys create a bit of historical déjà vu when they gather for the community roundup.

In the early 20th century, legends began to circulate about an enormous white wolf named Old Snowdrift whose mythical prowess and intelligence helped him evade trappers and wardens for years. Those who believed in his existence were rewarded when, in 1923, he and his mate were both caught. He was killed and his pelt put on display, but two of his pups were spared and shipped to Hollywood, where they starred on the silver screen for several years.

Set on a hillside above the creek, this campground is a place where RVs and tents peacefully coexist among a lodgepole pine, aspen, and Douglas-fir forest. Site 5 is the best for size and location, with plenty of room to spread out, a fair amount of privacy, and frontage on the creek. Site 6, across the road, is also on the creek, but it isn't as big. In general, sites are open, without a lot of overstory, but they are separated by thick undergrowth, and most have plenty of room for tents.

Hiking is the primary draw here. A well-connected network of trails winds through the creeks and ridges of the surrounding mountains. Most of the trails are open to horses, mountain bikes, and motorbikes (although visiting during the week should reduce your trail neighbors significantly). From the campground, Thain Creek Trail #411 is a short

Square Butte, east of the Highwood Mountains

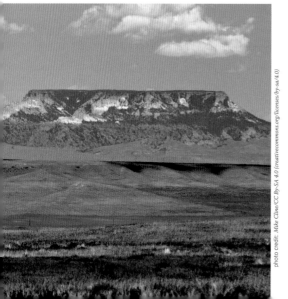

photo credit: Mike Cline/CC By-SA 4.0 (creativecommons.org/licenses/by-sa/4.0)

KEY INFORMATION

ADDRESS: Forest Road 8840, Great Falls, MT 59401

CONTACT: 406-566-2292; www.fs.usda.gov/helena

OPERATED BY: Helena–Lewis and Clark National Forest, Judith Ranger District

OPEN: Memorial Day weekend–mid-October; water available through Labor Day

SITES: 12

EACH SITE: Picnic table, fire ring

ASSIGNMENT: First come, first served; no reservations

REGISTRATION: On-site self-registration

FACILITIES: Water spigots, vault toilets

PARKING: At campsites

FEE: $5

ELEVATION: 4,520'

RESTRICTIONS:

Pets: On leash only

Fires: In fire rings only

Alcohol: Permitted

Vehicles: 30-foot length limit

Other: 16-day stay limit; pack in, pack out

0.75-mile loop combining the first section of Trail #411 with the final leg of Trail #431. This route is popular with kids, and there's plenty of room for them to explore. Another short trail is on Forest Road 8841, about a mile from the campground. This is a 1.5-mile environmental education trail with an accompanying interpretive brochure.

North Fork Highwood Creek Trail #423 lies west of the campground. Take FR 8840 south along the creek to the trailhead for this 14-mile out-and-back hike through meadows and along the river to its headwaters. The trail climbs 1,300 feet to the saddle before dropping to the Cottonwood Creek drainage, and the climb to the saddle is the only strenuous section. Combining Windy Mountain Trail #454 and Briggs Creek Trail #431 creates a 7-mile loop that climbs to a saddle south of Windy Mountain and then gently drops to a wildflower meadow. You'll encounter another saddle following Briggs Creek and then descend toward the trailhead.

A mile west on Forest Road 8830 is Highwoods Environmental Education Trail #452. This 1.5-mile interpretive trail is easy, informative, and for hikers only. Another nonmotorized option is Deer Creek Trail #453, off CR 121 southwest of the guard station. Although it doesn't actually make it to Highwood Baldy, this 3-mile out-and-back trail follows the creek and ends in a meadow from which a route along the ridge is possible.

Nearby as the crow flies are two significant geological features. To the northeast is Shonkin Sag, a 500-foot-deep, 1-mile-wide U-shaped valley that was cut by an ancient river draining glacial melt-off. Farther east, rising 2,500 feet above the plain, is Square Butte Natural Area. Visible for 100 miles across the eastern Montana plains, it was named "Fort Mountain" by Meriwether Lewis in 1805 and is featured in many of Charlie Russell's paintings.

Thain Creek Campground

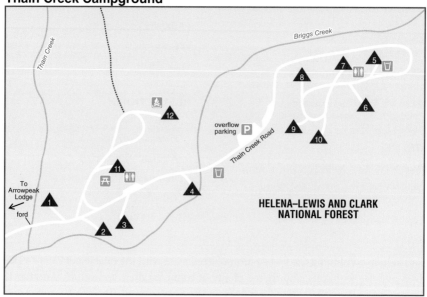

GETTING THERE

From Great Falls, take US 87/US 89 east for 6 miles to MT 228. Turn left and continue 13.9 miles on MT 228 to a stop sign. Go straight for 20 miles on the gravel road to the campground.

GPS COORDINATES: N47° 28.533' W110° 35.117'

21

Wood Lake Campground

Beauty: ★★★★★ / Privacy: ★★★★★ / Quiet: ★★★★ / Spaciousness: ★★★★ / Security: ★★★ /
Cleanliness: ★★★★★

Enjoy breathtaking scenery, a sparkling mountain lake, and access to miles of hiking in the Bob Marshall Wilderness Area.

Nestled in Wood Canyon, this campground offers dramatic mountain views to the north and rugged rock walls to the southwest. Except for breathtaking scenery, the sparkling mountain lake, and access to miles of hiking trails in the Bob Marshall Wilderness Area, you may find Wood Lake a little dull.

The campground lies along the eastern edge of the wilderness area, and since the parking areas and roadway are narrow, it's perfectly suited for tent camping. RVers head for nearby South Fork and Benchmark Campgrounds, which offer wider spaces. The campground is on the opposite side of the road from the lake, but it's only a short walk to the lakeshore. This is a place where you can expect to see wildlife and have long debates about which trail to hike.

This isn't a large or heavily wooded campground, but with fewer trees, the views extend in every direction. If privacy is important to you, site 7, on the outside edge of the loop, sits farthest from the road and is the quietest and most secluded spot. If you're traveling with another group, opt for sites 11 and 12, set off to the left before you get to the main loop.

You'll find brook, cutthroat, and rainbow trout in the lake, and if you decide not to fish, a lazy afternoon of canoeing will keep you near the water when the temperature rises. Deer, elk, and bears frequent the area, and many campers are lucky enough to see at least one of the peregrine falcons that nest here.

Drive to the parking area at Benchmark Campground, 6 miles farther west on Forest Service Road 235, to sit beside the creek on a mellow summer afternoon and watch the high mountain snowmelt cascade over boulders. This is Bob Marshall country: the Bob Marshall Wilderness Complex includes the Bob Marshall, Scapegoat, and Great Bear Wildernesses, totaling more than 1.5 million acres of trees, rivers, mountains, and wildlife in a wilderness preserved against the impact of progress and technology. You'll understand what Marshall meant when he wrote that wilderness is "the lapping of waves against the shoreline and the melody of wind in the trees."

Bob Marshall is the man responsible for developing the framework to protect this expansive pocket of Montana and others like it. He knew the area well, taking legendary day hikes of 30–70 miles that were more than simply a physical challenge; they intensified his passion for the wilderness—a passion that focused on preserving a place where everyone

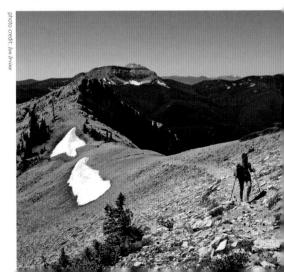

Wood Lake Campground provides access to several trails in the Bob Marshall Wilderness Area.

photo credit: Jon Irvine

KEY INFORMATION

ADDRESS: Benchmark Road
(Forest Road 235), Augusta, MT 59410

CONTACT: 406-466-5341,
www.fs.usda.gov/helena

OPERATED BY: Helena–Lewis and Clark
National Forest, Rocky Mountain
Ranger District

OPEN: Memorial Day–November,
weather permitting

SITES: 10 single sites and 2 double sites

EACH SITE: Picnic table, fire ring

ASSIGNMENT: First come, first served;
no reservations

REGISTRATION: On-site self-registration

FACILITIES: Hand-pump well, vault toilets

PARKING: At campsites

FEE: $6

ELEVATION: 5,500'

RESTRICTIONS:

Pets: On leash only

Fires: In fire ring only

Alcohol: Permitted

Vehicles: 35-foot length limit

Other: 16-day stay limit; pack in, pack out;
nonmotorized boats; bear-country food-
storage requirements

---

can experience days when the cycles of nature—not the hours on a clock—dictate the schedule.

Born and raised in New York City, Marshall was instrumental in expanding the country's fledgling wilderness system. In the late 1930s, as a division chief with the U.S. Forest Service, he singlehandedly brought more than 5 million acres under its protection. Two years after his untimely death at the age of 38, the Bob Marshall Wilderness area was formally designated and protected. "The Bob," as many Montanans affectionately call it, is a lasting legacy to the impact of one man's vision.

For those seeking something a bit shorter in distance, several options exist, but the closest are Wood Lake Trail #263, a short, easy stroll, and Patrol Mountain Trail #213, which begins just up the road. Trail #213 follows Straight Creek Trail for the first 3 miles, with refreshing creek crossings along the way. One particularly wide crossing is on Straight Creek, but when it's shallow it shouldn't be a problem. The trail then branches off for the final steady, steep 3-mile climb to a U.S. Forest Service lookout. This trail climbs just above 8,000 feet at the lookout, and you should expect to encounter some snow here and in Honeymoon Basin well into the early weeks of summer.

Petty Ford Creek Trail #244 begins 4 miles east of Wood Lake near Double Falls. It climbs briefly above Ford Creek and then gradually drops 400 feet over 3 miles to Petty Creek. You'll glimpse plenty of mountain views along the way, and you should have the trail pretty much to yourself. At Petty Creek you can continue on Smith Creek Trail #215 through the forests, with a few shallow creek crossings. This is a lightly traveled area, and you might have the waterfalls along the way all to yourself.

Wood Lake Campground

GETTING THERE

From Augusta, take Benchmark Road (FR 235) west for 24 miles to the campground.

GPS COORDINATES: N47° 25.667' W112° 47.600'

EASTERN MONTANA

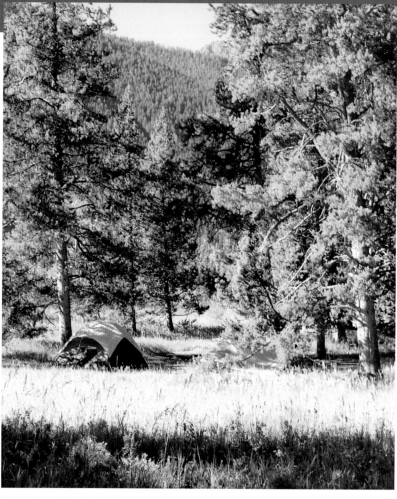

Beaver Creek County Park Campgrounds *(see next page)*

22

Beaver Creek County Park Campgrounds

Beauty: ★★★★ / Privacy: ★★★ / Quiet: ★★★★ / Spaciousness: ★★★★★ / Security: ★★★★ / Cleanliness: ★★★★

This 17-mile-long, 10,000-acre oasis straddles Beaver Creek.

Most people probably haven't heard of Fort Assinniboine, but when it was built in 1879 near the Milk River, it was the largest fort west of the Mississippi, encompassing all of the Bears Paw Mountains. The fort was built in response to concerns about Indian attacks after General Custer's defeat at Little Big Horn in 1876 and Chief Joseph's surrender in 1877 at Bear Paw Battlefield, 37 miles southeast. Before the fort was abandoned in 1911, General John Pershing served here as a lieutenant, and two companies of the 10th Cavalry "Buffalo Soldiers" trained here prior to their service in the Spanish-American War. Some of the fort's buildings still stand 6 miles southwest of Havre on US 87, and walking tours are available.

After the fort was abandoned, much of the land was designated as the Rocky Boy's Reservation, and the section that ultimately became Beaver Creek County Park bounced between the federal government, the state, and the city of Havre until it was finally established as a Hill County park in 1948.

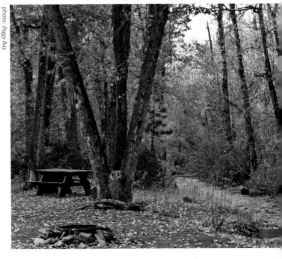

photo: Peggy Ray

In the thick of it, right next to Beaver Creek

Nestled on the northern edge of the Bears Paw Mountains, this park is an anomaly: it is possibly the country's largest county park but receives no county funds, and is set along a sparsely populated stretch of a state that, unlike many Midwestern and Eastern states, has very few county parks. Located in an island mountain range, where the highest peaks are generally buttes topping out around 5,000 feet, this is a 17-mile-long, 10,000-acre oasis that straddles Beaver Creek amid both vast areas of grasslands and groves of pines, cottonwoods, box elders, and willows that line the creek. It includes two large lakes and numerous feeder streams, and while there are no officially designated trails, bushwhacked trails are common. Geologists delight in the variety they find here, with glacial deposits in the northern section, volcanic evidence in the middle, and fossil-filled sedimentary cliffs in the south.

This is considered excellent terrain for ATVs and motorcycles, but they are banned from mid-May to mid-September and permitted only when the ground is frozen and snow-covered in winter; thus, there's plenty of room for hikers and mountain bikers. If you're driving the

KEY INFORMATION

ADDRESS: 17863 Beaver Creek Road, Havre, MT 59501

CONTACT: 406-395-4565, bcpark.org

OPERATED BY: Hill County Parks

OPEN: Year-round

SITES: 120–150

EACH SITE: Picnic table, fire grate, trash can

ASSIGNMENT: First come, first served; reservations accepted at largest sites

REGISTRATION: Purchase daily and annual passes at the park office or from vendors in Havre (see website)

FACILITIES: Water available at park office, vault toilets, boat launch

PARKING: At campsites

FEE: $10/day, $30–$70/year depending on age and residence

ELEVATION: 3,171'–4,113'

RESTRICTIONS:

Pets: On leash only

Fires: In fire rings only

Alcohol: Permitted

Vehicles: No length restrictions, though access roads could be a problem for longer vehicles

Other: 14-day stay limit per campsite

park road, you probably won't notice it, but if you're on a bicycle, you'll definitely feel the nearly 1,000-foot elevation gain from the north end to the south end of the park.

Within the park you'll find about two dozen different camping areas, in addition to group sites, picnic areas, and a youth camp. The superintendent's office isn't sure how many campsites exist, as sites within designated campgrounds are not always well defined. Each campground has vault toilets, and several have shelters that can be reserved.

Daily and annual passes are available at the park office (adjacent to the youth camp) or at vendors in town. Daily passes are also available at two self-pay boxes: one by the RV dump site in the middle of the park and another near the information kiosk at the north entrance.

Beaver Creek is heavily used by local residents and those traveling the Hi-Line, but there always seems to be room for one more camper. (The Hi-Line is an area extending across northern Montana that follows US 2 and the east–west railroad tracks originally laid by the Great Northern Railway in the 1800s.) Fishing is

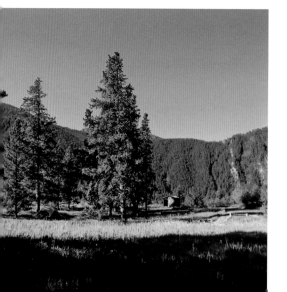

Like that spot? It's yours! Not all sites at Beaver Creek are well defined.

excellent, with rainbow and brook trout stocked at both lakes and in Beaver Creek, while Lower Beaver Creek Lake also offers anglers the opportunity to land perch, northern pike, and walleyes. The park is also a wildlife watcher's paradise, ripe with white-tailed and mule deer, as well as eagles, hawks, bobcats, and several areas where beavers create intricate dams.

At the south end of the park is access to the Rocky Boy's Indian Reservation, thousands of rolling acres owned by the Chippewa Cree tribe. The tribe holds its annual powwow each August, and the public is invited to view and participate in a variety of cultural demonstrations and try a full menu of traditional foods.

Life in Montana, particularly along the Hi-Line, can be hard, and adaptability is crucial. Business owners in Havre proved their flexibility when a January 1904 fire destroyed most of the town, and they simply moved their establishments underground until reconstruction could begin. Today, places like Sporting Eagle Saloon, a Chinese laundry, and an opium den have been restored to their early 1900s appearance, and guided tours are given.

The town of Havre, one of the Great Northern Railway's original stops, still serves as a stop for Amtrak trains headed to Chicago, Seattle, and Portland. Train lovers will want to stop at the city's railroad museum and spend some time chatting with the volunteers, whose knowledge and stories are a delight.

Beaver Creek County Park Campgrounds

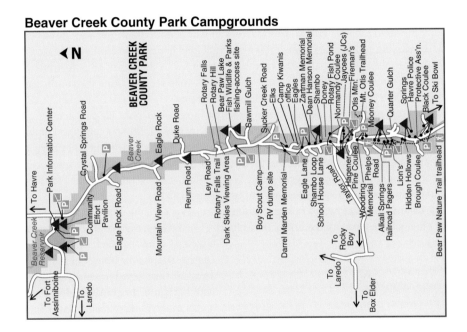

GETTING THERE

From Havre, take Beaver Creek Road south for 10 miles to the first campground, at the northern end of Beaver Creek Park.

GPS COORDINATES: N48° 24.666' W109° 43.046'

23

⛺ Camp Creek Campground

Beauty: ★★★★ / Privacy: ★★★★ / Quiet: ★★★★★ / Spaciousness: ★★★★ / Security: ★★★★ /
Cleanliness: ★★★★★

The forest surrounding Camp Creek is an unexpected surprise in this region of vast plains and few trees.

Camp Creek sits in a quiet pocket of the Little Rocky Mountains, an island range that rises not to massive heights with steep exposed crags like its western siblings but to softer, undulating heights peppered with thick timber and sections of igneous rock. These mountains, which the Gros Ventre tribe call the Fur Caps, were a sacred area for vision quests before the intrusion of gold fever. When the Fort Belknap Indian Reservation was originally designated, it included the area around Camp Creek; it would not remain this way, however. By 1895, trespassing prospectors knew there were rich gold deposits beneath the surface, and the native people were no match for a growing nation fed by dreams of great fortunes. The federal government "negotiated" the sale of a 7- by 4-mile section along the south-central border for $360,000, sealing the deal with a revised treaty.

Within this tiny section lay a mother lode that miners had been illegally accessing for years, and after the 1895 treaty, the mining furor increased. Prospector Pike Landusky struck it rich but was killed in his own saloon by outlaw and local resident Kid Curry. Pete Zortman established his mill and the town that bears his name, and soon miners were extracting more than $10,000 of gold a day. World War I and several fires impeded things a bit, but the mines were not totally closed until the mid-1930s.

The historic mining town of Zortman still remains, just down the road from Camp Creek, and is often referred to as a ghost town. In reality, this is a thriving, close-knit community with a general store that serves as information central. Despite the impact of mining, this area still has beautiful mountains filled with big game, songbirds, eagles, coyotes, and beavers. Camp Creek is unexpectedly nestled in the trees and is often used by those seeking an overnight stop as they explore the Hi-Line region of the state, which extends across northern Montana following US 2 and the east–west railroad tracks originally laid by the Great Northern Railway in the 1800s.

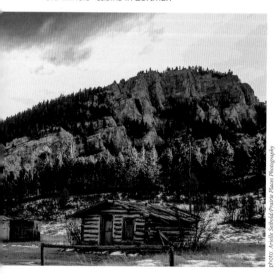

Old miners' cabins in Zortman

photo: Arielle Seibold/Prairie Places Photography

Sites here vary from perfect for tenters to a few that offer no place to pitch a tent except for the gravel RV pull-through pad. The first six sites on the loop road have covered picnic tables, and sites 1 and 2 are across the road from a nice pair of horseshoe pits. Site 5 is the

KEY INFORMATION

ADDRESS: Bear Gulch Road, Malta, MT 59538

CONTACT: 406-654-5100, blm.gov

OPERATED BY: Bureau of Land Management, Malta Field Office

OPEN: Year-round depending on weather conditions; full services May–September

SITES: 20 (13 in main loop)

EACH SITE: Picnic table, fire grate

ASSIGNMENT: First come, first served; no reservations

REGISTRATION: On-site self-registration

FACILITIES: Water spigots, drinking fountains, vault toilets, group areas, bearproof trash cans

PARKING: At campsites

FEE: $10

ELEVATION: 3,500'

RESTRICTIONS:

Pets: On leash only

Fires: In fire rings only

Alcohol: Permitted

Vehicles: No restrictions

Other: 14-day stay limit; bear-country food storage restrictions

---

most private, with dense understory and plenty of room for a pair of tents. Sites 8 and 9 accommodate tents but offer little privacy, and sites 7, 10, and 11 have no tent area at all.

A designated auto-tour route through the Charles M. Russell National Wildlife Refuge begins 37 miles south on US 191. This 19-mile driving tour stops at 13 interpretive points, and it takes a minimum of 2 hours to travel. The gravel roads provide excellent access to unspoiled Missouri Breaks scenery and wildlife viewing. This land remains close to what it was like when Lewis and Clark saw it in 1805, and it offers the vistas that artist Charles M. Russell loved best. Plan to stop along the way and explore by hiking off the main roads. You won't see the wealth of bison or bighorn sheep that the Corps of Discovery saw or the grizzly bears and wolves that plagued early homesteaders, but there are dozens of other mammals and over 200 bird species, which makes a bird guide a welcome companion. Campers are advised to practice "bear aware" behavior, as black bears periodically visit the area, including the campground, which resulted in the installation of bearproof trash cans in 2016.

The Missouri River to the west of the refuge is designated as a part of the National Wild and Scenic River System, and much of the land along both sides, from the refuge to Coal Banks Landing, was designated as the Upper Missouri River Breaks National Monument in 2001. If you have a canoe, this is a spectacular stretch of river. But be sure to contact the Bureau of Land Management in Lewistown for the most current regulations.

The sign says it all.

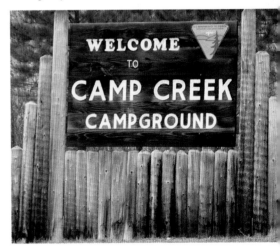

To the northwest is Bear Paw Battlefield, part of the Nez Perce National Historical Park. This is where the last battle of the Nez Perce War of 1877 was fought and where Nez Perce Chief Joseph finally surrendered. The museum in Chinook serves as a visitor center, and there is a self-guided interpretive trail at the battlefield.

During your visit to Camp Creek, you may still see evidence of the impact of mining. It is estimated that billions of dollars worth of gold was extracted here in the 20th century, more than $300 million of that from the 1970s to the 1990s. All of this came from a piece of land that cost the United States $360,000 to purchase in 1895, but it may cost well over $40 million to partially clean up.

Camp Creek Campground

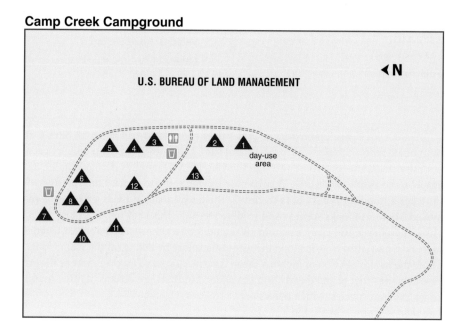

GETTING THERE

From Malta, take US 191 south for 40 miles to Bear Gulch Road. Turn right and go 8 miles east to the campground sign. Turn right and go 1 mile north to the campground.

GPS COORDINATES: N47° 55.487' W108° 30.247'

24

Crystal Lake Campground

Beauty: ★★★★★ / Privacy: ★★★★★ / Quiet: ★★★★ / Spaciousness: ★★★★★ / Security: ★★★★★ /
Cleanliness: ★★★★

Hiking trails abound in this pristine setting.

Crystal Lake is different from most high-mountain lakes. It's very shallow, about 13 feet deep in the spring after the mountain snowmelt, and by the end of the summer it may dwindle to only 5 feet. The lake's water gradually seeps out through its porous limestone bottom until it is almost nonexistent, and then the snowmelt begins again. As a result, the trout found here are restocked annually, since they can't survive the thick ice cover and lack of oxygen in the winter. The lake is perfect for canoes and float tubes and attracts family groups.

The limestone cliffs you'll see were formed about 350,000 years ago, and fossils are visible in many of them. Also along the cliffs you may see one of the resident mountain goats or the nests of golden eagles or prairie falcons. The mountain goats are not natives, since this island range is too far from their home in the western parts of the state, but they were transported here in 1954 and have adapted well to the Big Snowy Mountains. The range lives up to its name, with peaks that top out above 8,000 feet and are usually snowcapped well into July. The Big Snowies are often called a laboratory range, due to continued geological study of the formation's 400-million-year history and wealth of visible fossils. Hikers and campers may come across fossils or notice the sedimentary aspects, but their appreciation is generally for the recreational aspects of this distinctive island in the midst of the prairies.

Finding a site on summer weekends is a challenge, since there aren't many established campgrounds in this section of the state. When the weather is nice, it often appears that everyone is heading out to camp and hike. Some fairly large RVs manage to navigate the access road, but you'll find several tenters in the mix, and there is enough understory that you may not even be aware of your neighbors. Campsites here are well spaced and roomy, with plenty of privacy. None is actually lakeside, and the foliage that cre-

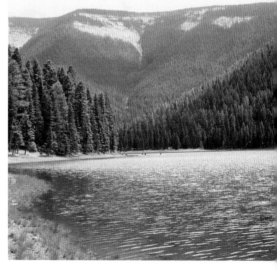

Crystal Lake is sheltered by the Big Snowy Mountains.

ates cozy, private sites also provides a good buffer against hikers on the shoreline trail. Sites 7, 21, and 24 are the largest and most secluded, while sites 16, 17, and 18 are quiet and well hidden by spruce trees. Access to the shoreline loop trail is next to site 4, making it the least private, but it still isn't too bad. The group site is very popular for family reunions, and reservations are required for groups.

KEY INFORMATION

ADDRESS: Crystal Lake Road, Lewistown, MT 59457

CONTACT: 406-566-2292, www.fs.usda.gov/helena

OPERATED BY: Helena–Lewis and Clark National Forest, Judith Ranger District

OPEN: Mid-June–September, depending on the weather

SITES: 28, plus group area

EACH SITE: Picnic table, fire grate

ASSIGNMENT: First come, first served; reservations for group area only

REGISTRATION: On-site self-registration; group area must be reserved by calling 877-444-6777 or visiting recreation.gov.

FACILITIES: Water spigots, vault toilets, boat launch

PARKING: At campsites

FEE: $10

ELEVATION: 5,700'

RESTRICTIONS:

Pets: On leash only

Fires: In fire rings only

Alcohol: Permitted

Vehicles: 35-foot length limit

Other: 16-day stay limit; bear-country food storage restrictions; pack in, pack out; nonmotorized watercraft only in the lake

---

Hiking options from this campground may offer the most variety found in a single area in the state. The easiest hike is the Shoreline Loop Trail #404, a 1.75-mile loop marked with interpretive posts that correspond to the informational brochure available from the campground host. From the Loop Trail you can access the 0.5-mile Wildflower Trail, where most wildflowers bloom in July and August.

Another moderate hike is Crystal Cascades Trail #445, which leads to a delightful waterfall, where the water drops from a cave down stair-step ledges for nearly 100 feet. This trail can be combined with others for an 8-mile-loop day hike.

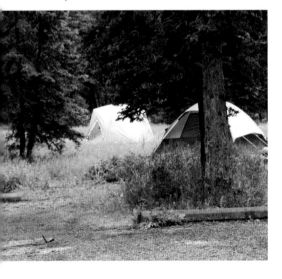

Tenters enjoying the peace in a secluded meadow at Crystal Lake.

If your goal is to hit some mountain peaks, take Trail #403 to Grandview Point and West Peak. It's 3.5 miles to Grandview Point, with forest and vista views along the way. From there you'll enjoy a panoramic view of Crystal Lake and the entire Judith Basin. Another 1.5 miles takes you along a ridge to West Peak, one of the highest ridges in the Snowy Range.

For something different, try the 5-mile hike to the Ice Caves. The trailhead for this hike is at the parking lot and leads to permanent ice caves high atop the ridge. To get there, you'll climb 2,200 feet over 3 miles to the top of Snowy Crest and then follow an open ridge marked by cairns for another 2 miles. The view on a clear day extends to the Teton Mountains in Wyoming (220 miles south). You'll be at about

8,000 feet on both this hike and the Grandview/West hike, so don't be surprised if you still see snow in June and even early July.

A wealth of additional hiking trails crisscrosses the range, and many are well suited for mountain bikers. Neil Creek Trail #654 branches off near the ice caves, and bikers frequently see black bears along the creek near the trailhead. Horses share most trails with mountain bikers and hikers, but practicing good trail ethics and using common sense will provide a memorable experience for everyone.

Crystal Lake Campground

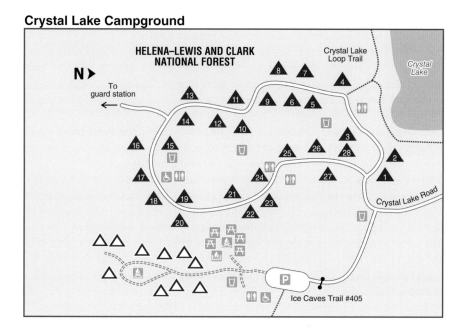

GETTING THERE

From Lewistown, take US 87 west for 8.7 miles to Crystal Lake Road. Turn left and go 5.3 miles to a Y intersection. Bear left and go 3.9 miles to the recreation-area sign. Turn left at the sign, continuing on Crystal Lake Road, and go 12.7 miles to the campground.

From Harlowton, take US 191 north for 35.5 miles to Sipple Road. Turn right and go 21.5 miles to the campground, following the signs for Crystal Lake Recreation Area. The road to the campground varies from narrow two-lane to single-lane and from dirt to paved.

GPS COORDINATES: N46° 47.633' W109° 30.667'

25

Makoshika State Park Campground

Beauty: ★★★★★ / Privacy: ★★★ / Quiet: ★★★★★ / Spaciousness: ★★★ / Security: ★★★★★ /
Cleanliness: ★★★★★

Explore this geological and paleontological time capsule.

The Lakota Sioux called this the "Land of Bad Spirits." Mushroom-shaped cap rocks, flat-topped buttes, spires pointing skyward, razor-sharp hogbacks, and fluted hillsides combine to create a land of curious formations shaped by wind and water.

But wait a minute, you think, as you drive through the neighborhood in Glendive that borders the park entrance, this looks like typical, middle-of-nowhere, safe and friendly small-town America. Where is the dramatic landscape of "bad spirits," and what's with those dinosaur tracks on the street? When does the gigantic monster come plodding along to destroy the innocent townies?

Even after you enter the park and arrive at the visitor center, this description will seem more fiction than fact, but just keep driving. A stop at the center will give you an overall view of the park and its history, taking you on a multimillion-year journey.

Tenters will want to bypass the 15-unit lower campground and continue another 1.5 miles up the paved road to Pine on Rocks Campground, Cap Rock Campground, or Valley View Campground. Take your time while driving, and don't be fooled: this road is steep (a 15-percent grade in some sections), and the switchbacks enforce a slow speed.

The nine rustic tent sites in these three areas are tucked into a precious oasis of hard-to-find shade, and they are rarely full, because most visitors don't realize they exist. It isn't entirely primitive: there are fire rings, picnic tables, and a vault toilet. Water is available only at the visitor center, though.

So have you noticed anything yet? Something like a slight change in the landscape? Surreal, isn't it? Mother Nature has carved herself a beauty here, with wind-chiseled sandstone to your left and thick stands of pine and junipers to your right. It has taken a few years, actually about 70 million, for this 11,500-acre park to look like this. In the early 1900s,

Makoshika State Park: it's otherworldly.

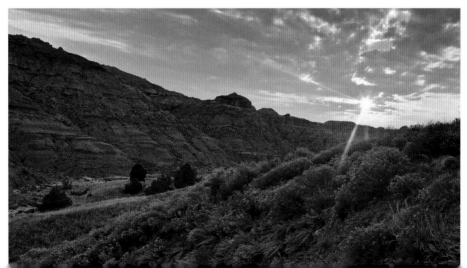

KEY INFORMATION

ADDRESS: 1301 Snyder Ave., Glendive, MT 59330

CONTACT: 406-377-6256 or 406-234-0900, stateparks.mt.gov/makoshika; reservations: reserveamerica.com

OPERATED BY: Makoshika State Park

OPEN: May–September

SITES: 24, including 9 dispersed rustic sites

EACH SITE: Picnic table, fire grate

ASSIGNMENT: First come, first served or by reservation

REGISTRATION: On-site self-registration or online

FACILITIES: Water spigot at visitor center only, vault toilets, interpretive center, nature trails, scenic drive, amphitheater, disc golf course

PARKING: At campsites

FEE: $12 rustic resident, $18 standard resident, $28 nonresident; $6/extra nonresident vehicle

ELEVATION: 2,374'

RESTRICTIONS:

Pets: On leash only

Fires: In fire rings only

Alcohol: Permitted

Vehicles: No length limit at lower campground; tents only at rustic sites

Other: 14-day stay limit

it was promoted as a potential national park. Thankfully, this prehistoric seabed didn't make the cut, and it remains uncrowded and minimally developed. In addition, it has evolved as a paleontologist's dream, where bones from former residents named *Triceratops, Edmontosaurus, Tyrannosaurus rex*, and *Thescelosaurus* protrude and ancient plant and sea life fossils dot the ground, revealing themselves to the patient observer.

If you're lucky enough to find something, don't take it or disturb it. Feel free to take photographs, and be sure to inform the visitor center staff of your find and its location. Who knows? You may have stumbled onto an entirely unknown species that could someday be named after its discoverer—you!

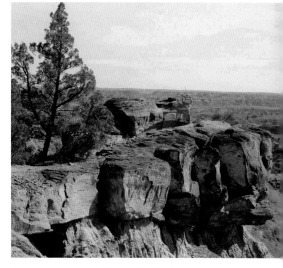

A rock outcrop near Pine-on-Rocks Campground at Makoshika

It's hard to believe as you look across the stark landscape that this was once a lush, semi-tropical environment similar to that found in Louisiana. Everything seems so dry, brown, and dull. But closer inspection reveals a wealth of color, with bands of red, pink, and yellow providing a backdrop for the evergreens and silvery sagebrush. Early morning and dusk provide endless possibilities to experience vibrant sunrises and sunsets, and photographers could spend days taking photos of the sandstone formations from different angles and in different weather.

The weather here provides contrasts as dramatic as the landscape itself. Ever-present winds flapping your tent walls are the same winds that continue to erode the rocks. Rain, which comes infrequently and often lasts only minutes, awakens dry riverbeds and occasionally causes torrents of water to rush through. Like adding water to dry cake mix, the soil becomes thick and heavy quickly, attaching to tires and shoes in large, gooey globs Montanans affectionately call "gumbo." On top of all this, there's the heat. Temperature extremes can be tremendous, shifting the thermometer 50 degrees in a few hours.

Within this dynamic area, wildflowers, including lupines, locoweed, prickly pear cactus, Indian paintbrush, yucca, and echinacea provide bold pockets of color. Coulees conceal deer, mountain lions, foxes, and coyotes. Sagebrush and grass provide cover for rabbits, bobcats, porcupines, and skunks and the sparse trees and gnarled snags are home to prairie falcons, red-tailed hawks, and golden eagles. Turkey vultures even make an annual pilgrimage, putting on a show by soaring high above the badlands and roosting in trees.

Throughout the park are vista points and picnic areas, an amphitheater, and a dozen trails ranging from short nature walks to longer backcountry routes. The unimproved road climbs and twists into the park's outer reaches, and along the way you'll see prairie rattlesnakes, which necessitate caution while hiking.

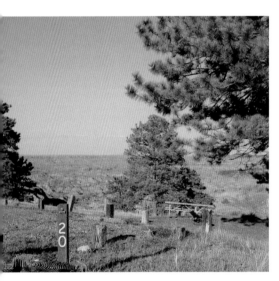

With a view like this, it's easy to spot dinosaurs before they spot you!

Camping here is unlike anything else Montana has to offer. Although it's out of the way for anyone who isn't traveling through the eastern part of the state, it's a unique opportunity to experience a geological and paleontological time capsule that has been virtually untouched for millions of years.

Makoshika State Park Campground

GETTING THERE

From Glendive, take Snyder Avenue southeast for 0.25 miles, or follow the hadrosaur tracks to the park.

GPS COORDINATES: N47° 5.383' W104° 42.380'

26

⛺ Sage Creek Campground

Beauty: ★★★★ / Privacy: ★★★★★ / Quiet: ★★★★★ / Spaciousness: ★★★★ / Security: ★★★ /
Cleanliness: ★★★★★

Bird-watching along Sage Creek may add sage thrashers, rock wrens, ruby-crowned kinglets, and warblers to your life list.

In the words of Chief Arapooish, "The Crow Country is a good country. The Great Spirit has put it in exactly the right place. While you are in it, you fare well; whenever you go out of it, whichever way you may travel, you fare worse." Sage Creek is perched near the heart of the Pryor Mountains in a landscape that is sacred to the Crow (Apsáalooke) tribe.

The home of another Crow leader, Chief Plenty Coups, is preserved as a state park, in Pryor. As a young man, Plenty Coups retreated to the Pryor Mountains for a vision quest, during which he foresaw the coming of the white people who would take his tribe's land. He told his people, "Education is your most powerful weapon. With education you are the white man's equal; without education you are his victim." Throughout his life, Plenty Coups traveled extensively. He met with leaders and politicians and was instrumental in accomplishing something rare: the designation of his tribe's homelands as their reservation. He was also selected to represent all Indians at the 1921 dedication of the Tomb of the Unknown Soldier in Arlington National Cemetery. He laid his war bonnet and coup stick at the memorial and prayed "that there will be peace to all men hereafter."

Thanks to a facelift by the U.S. Forest Service, Sage Creek is no longer a barren, forlorn place. Although there was nothing they could do to change the intense summer heat, the new design does address the lack of shade. New plantings of green ash, ponderosa pine, and cottonwoods help mitigate the fact that trees are hard to come by out here. Shade screens over each picnic table help as well. All campsites have been moved up on a rise, away from the creek. This reduced the mosquito problem dramatically and will allow the regeneration of riparian plants to preserve the stream channel and improve fish habitat. The vibrant sunsets and cool morning sunrises that you'll enjoy from your campsite are

Sage Creek Campgrounds is nestled "way out there" in the Pryor Mountains.

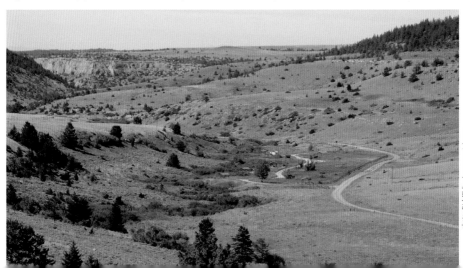

photo: *Dick Walton/pryormountains.org*

KEY INFORMATION

ADDRESS: Sage Creek Road, Bridger, MT 59014

CONTACT: 406-446-2103; www.fs.usda.gov/custergallatin

OPERATED BY: Custer Gallatin National Forest, Beartooth Ranger District

OPEN: Year-round when accessible; full services Memorial Day weekend–Labor Day

SITES: 10 (8 single, 2 double)

EACH SITE: Picnic table, fire ring

ASSIGNMENT: First come, first served; no reservations

REGISTRATION: On-site self-registration

FACILITIES: Water spigots (intermittently available; call ahead or bring your own water), vault toilets

PARKING: At campsites

FEE: $5

ELEVATION: 5,520'

RESTRICTIONS:

Pets: On leash only

Fires: In fire rings only

Alcohol: Permitted

Vehicles: 30-foot length limit

Other: 16-day stay limit; bear-country food storage restrictions; pack in, pack out

among the best in the state. With the new design, the possibility of having an RV for a neighbor may increase, but the rough road and small number of visitors to the Pryor Mountains still work in your favor.

The Pryor Mountains are one of the most ecologically diverse areas in Montana, offering ten different biological systems, from high desert to subalpine meadows. Rare plant species can be observed here, including bladderpod and *Shoshonea pulvinata.* The full range of large mammals—black bears, bighorn sheep, mule deer, and the occasional elk—make it a wildlife-watcher's paradise. Bird-watching along Sage Creek may add sage thrashers, rock wrens, ruby-crowned kinglets, and warblers to your wildlife list, and don't be surprised if a hummingbird or green-tailed towhee visits camp.

If you drive south on Pryor Creek Road, turn left at Warren and head east for about 20 miles on the designated gravel road. You'll arrive at the Pryor Mountain National Wild Horse Range. This is a dusty, sweltering drive in the dead of summer, but the dramatic canyons and chance that you might see one of the family groups that make up the herd is worth it.

Twelve miles east of Sage Creek on Forest Road 2308 is an amazing geological feature in the heart of the Pryor Mountains. Throughout the year, whether it's December or July, huge icicles form in this cave and the floor is coated with ice. Here at the creatively named Big Ice Cave, all characteristics for a natural deep freeze converge. In winter, cold air flows into the steep cave, forming ice on the floor and walls. In warmer months, the denser cold air sinks, the lighter warm air traps the cold air in the cave chamber, and the cycle continues, perpetuating the deep-freeze environment.

Don't expect a guided tour or extensive interpretive signs; the only development here is the walkway to the entrance and an interior viewing platform. Take a jacket—it's cold enough inside to keep ice frozen—and experience one of Mother Nature's refrigerators. While exploring the area, keep your eyes open for bats. Nearly a dozen species call the Pryors home; see if you can spot the differences between them.

If you continue up the road past the cave, you'll come to Dry Head Vista, where the view extends to Wyoming and the Big Horn Mountains. From here you can hike into Lost Water

Canyon, where you may spot some 200-million-year-old fossils, along with a variety of birds and plants, and maybe even a few members of the wild-horse herd.

Sage Creek Campground

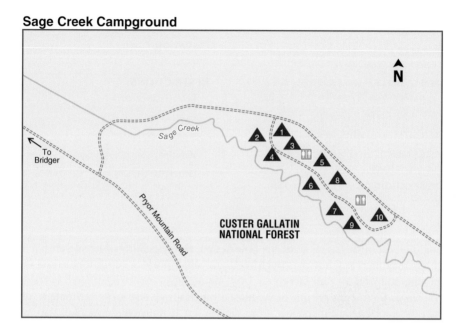

GETTING THERE

From the town of Bridger, go south 3 miles on US 310 to Pryor Mountain Road. Turn left, and within 2 miles the asphalt turns to gravel at the railroad crossing. Continue on good gravel for about 12 miles to a T junction, where you turn right. Travel for about 3 miles to another T junction, where you turn left. On a narrowing gravel road, in about 5 miles, you arrive at Sage Creek Road, where you turn right following Sage Creek. In nearly 5 more miles, turn left and cross the creek, and go 1 mile to the campground. Note that some of these roads are gravel and dirt and can be rutted or become impassable in wet weather.

GPS COORDINATES: N45° 12.833' W108° 33.278'

SOUTH CENTRAL MONTANA

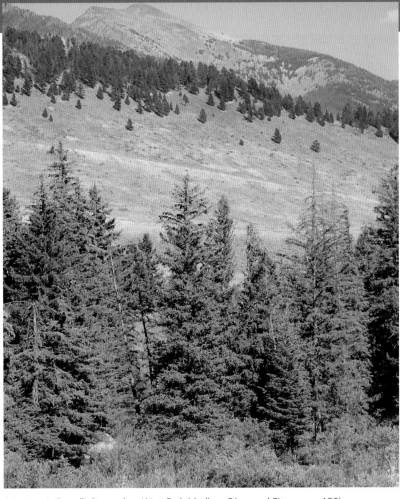

Montana's Gravelly Range *(see West Fork Madison Dispersed Sites, page 130)*

Battle Ridge Campground

Beauty: ★★★★ / Privacy: ★★★ / Quiet: ★★★★ / Spaciousness: ★★★★ / Security: ★★★★ /
Cleanliness: ★★★★

For campers geared up with boots and a mountain bike, the rewards reached from the campground are numerous.

In 1878, near the site of this campground, a battle between American Indians and cowboys over horses ended the life of one cowboy. Consequently, the skirmish provided the name for Battle Ridge Pass and the campground, both of which could easily be named today for peace and beauty—or wildflowers.

The campground sits on a slight tilt toward the west, providing a splendid view of the Bridger Mountains, a north–south subrange of the Rocky Mountains with a serpentine ridgeline. Bozeman Pass, located on I-90 between Livingston and Bozeman, separates the Bridger Range from the Gallatin Mountains, distinguishing the southern edge of this range, named after mountain man Jim Bridger. Clinging to the eastside slopes of the range, Bridger Bowl Ski Area is located about 5 miles south of the campground, or 16 miles from Bozeman.

In the fair-weather months, the mountain range is synonymous with activities such as hiking, climbing, wildlife viewing, mountain biking, and a 20-mile foot race, the Bridger Ridge Run, routed along the ridgeline from Fairy Lake at the north to the "M" at the southern end. The campground attracts enthusiasts who enjoy these pursuits and offers a peaceful respite for travelers who enjoy exploring secondary routes through Montana.

In spite of the highway intercepting the western view, the sites are heaven for tenters, with small parking spaces (deterring large RVs), a fire ring, picnic tables,

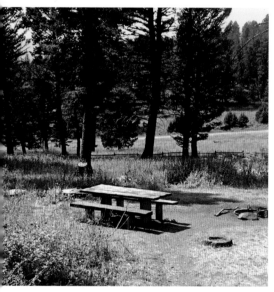

Battle Ridge Campground: simple, peaceful, and smack-dab in the middle of a mountain playground

and comfortable spaces for tents. Sites 1–9 are upslope, farther from the highway—traffic is rarely heavy and ebbs by dusk.

For campers geared up with boots and a mountain bike, the rewards reached from the campground are numerous.

You can easily spend days here exploring the area, hiking trails, climbing summits, and mountain biking. For a kick-off, try the moderate 2-mile (one-way) hike to Ross Pass on the Ross Pass Connector Trail #551. To get to the trailhead, drive a mile north of the campground and turn left at Brackett Creek onto FR 631. Drive the old logging road for about

KEY INFORMATION

ADDRESS: MT 86, Bozeman, MT 59718

CONTACT: 406-522-2520, www.fs.usda.gov /custergallatin

OPERATED BY: Custer Gallatin National Forest, Bozeman Ranger District

OPEN: Whenever accessible, mainly May–September

SITES: 13

EACH SITE: Picnic table, fire ring

ASSIGNMENT: First come, first served; no reservations

REGISTRATION: On-site self-registration

FACILITIES: Vault toilets but no drinking water

PARKING: At campsites

FEE: Free

ELEVATION: 6,500'

RESTRICTIONS:

Pets: On leash only

Fires: In fire rings only

Alcohol: Permitted

Vehicles: 1 vehicle/site; 30-foot length limit

Other: 16-day stay limit; bear-country food storage restrictions; no firewood or water; pack in, pack out

3 miles to the trailhead. Sections of the primitive road are tricky to drive without a high-clearance vehicle. The hiking trail ascends gradually until it steepens on the final push to the pass.

Even before you step into the open meadow at the pass, you will notice the impressive crag to the north. You're at the high foot of Ross Peak, the fourth highest summit in the Bridger Range. Climbing to its 9,003-foot summit requires scrambling skills over steep and rocky terrain and, while not overly technical, requires more than an ounce of courage for some folks. You game?

If not, try Sacajawea Peak. The range's highest mountain (9,838') asks only for hiking skills to summit. Sacajawea Peak Trail #509 is located at Fairy Lake, which is also the location of Fairy Lake Campground and its 9 campsites. To get there, drive the highway about 2 miles north of the Battle Ridge Campground and turn left (west) onto Fairy Lake Road (Forest Road 74) and continue for 5 miles on an intermittently rough, steep gravel road. A high-clearance vehicle is recommended.

The 2-mile trail to the summit begins on switchbacks and then levels through an alpine valley before leading you up another, longer series of switchbacks to a saddle. Turn left (east) directly toward the summit, avoiding the Bridger Foothills National Recreation Trail heading south, and ascend the trail. Near to or on the summit, you could see mountain goats. They're common near the summit, where you will encounter impressive views of the Bridger Range, the Gallatin Valley, and, to the east, the Crazy Mountains and the Shields River Valley. To the northwest, you will see Hardscrabble Peak (9,575'), the Bridger Range's second highest peak, and a tantalizing line to its summit. It is easily accessed from the saddle separating the two mountains, which compels many climbers to bag both peaks in a day.

For mountain bikers, the Bangtail Divide Trail #504 is a prized singletrack sure to dazzle. The ridgeline traverse offers excellent loop or out-and-back options through fields of wildflowers, with superb views of mountain ranges east and west. Get to the action by driving

Bridger Canyon Road south of Battle Ridge for about 7 miles, passing Bridger Bowl and turning left (east) on Stone Creek Road. Travel the gravel road to a parking area just before a gate. The other access is the Bracket Creek trailhead, about a mile north of the campground.

Battle Ridge Campground

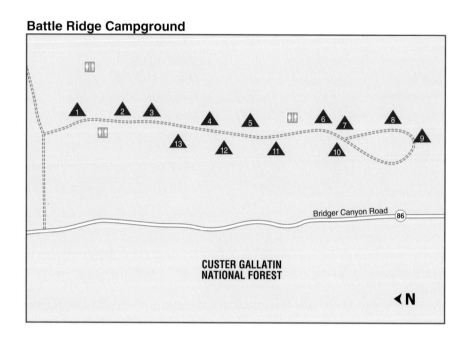

GETTING THERE

From Bozeman, take MT 86 (Bridger Canyon Road) north for 22 miles and turn right into the campground.

GPS COORDINATES: N45° 52.892' W110° 52.810'

28

Beaver Creek Campground

Beauty: ★★★★★ / Privacy: ★★★ / Quiet: ★★★★ / Spaciousness: ★★★★★ / Security: ★★★★★ /
Cleanliness: ★★★★★

Placid mountain views and the sparkling waters of Quake Lake draw many to this spot.

Montana is a land of contrasts formed by the continuous shifting of the earth, and on August 17, 1959, the Madison River Valley was where it chose to tremble and shake. During that brief moment, which by geologic time is nearly immeasurable, 80 million tons of mountainside slid from its perch, causing a brief but massive windstorm. Before the dust settled, a river was rerouted and a new lake was formed. It was a cataclysmic geologic event, and it was over in an instant.

For the people in the Madison River Valley, however, this nanosecond of geologic time seemed to last forever. Violently awakened on what had been a calm, star-filled night, hundreds of campers, tourists, and residents found themselves in a confusing and disorienting chaos. Twenty-eight people were killed by the quake's power. Nineteen were buried alive under the massive landslide.

It has been nearly 60 years since the disaster, and a visit to this valley is still humbling. The barren mountainside remains, and absorbing the enormity and suddenness of the event leaves one feeling insignificant and helpless against the forces Mother Nature can unleash.

The same forces of nature that created chaos in 1959 are also responsible for the immense, stark beauty and sense of peace found here today. Placid mountain views and the sparkling water of Quake Lake draw many to this spot halfway between historic Virginia City and Yellowstone National Park.

Quake Lake

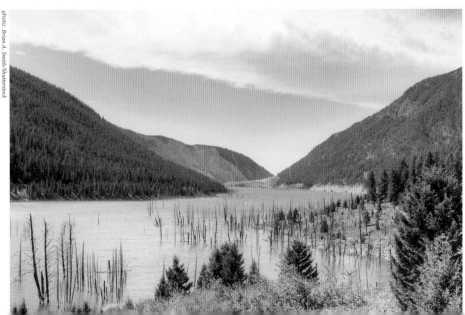

photo: *Brian A. Smith/Shutterstock*

KEY INFORMATION

ADDRESS: Hebgen Lake Road (US 287), West Yellowstone, MT 59758

CONTACT: 406-823-6961, www.fs.usda.gov /custergallatin; reservations: 877-444-6777, recreation.gov

OPERATED BY: Custer Gallatin National Forest, Hebgen Lake Ranger District

OPEN: Late May–September 30

SITES: 63

EACH SITE: Picnic table, fire grate

ASSIGNMENT: First come, first served or by reservation

REGISTRATION: On-site self-registration

FACILITIES: Water spigots, vault toilets; interpretive center 4 miles away

PARKING: At campsites

FEE: $15

ELEVATION: 6,500'

RESTRICTIONS:

Pets: On leash only

Fires: In fire rings only

Alcohol: Permitted

Vehicles: 32-foot length limit

Other: 16-day stay limit; bear-country food storage restrictions

A long entry road into the campground provides a buffer from the noise on the highway, creating a sense of isolation. The campground is divided into three loops and offers numerous tenting options. The entry road splits, and to the left is Loop A, with beautiful mountain views to the south. A mix of lodgepole pine and aspen divide the spacious sites here. The road drops downhill as you round the backside of the loop, offering additional privacy for sites A4–A9.

Sites A7 and A8 are near a beaver pond. A8 is the better choice, thanks to a good view of the mountains and more room for a tent. Early in the season these sites might have standing water, making mosquitoes a problem. A10 is the prime site on this loop. You'll need to be a little creative in situating your tent, but you'll have great morning sun and you'll be at the back of the loop, secluded from most of the other sites.

To the right, off the entrance road, is Loop B, and Loop C continues straight ahead. Loop B is heavily forested; Site B5, on the inside of the loop, is perfect for a larger group. Site B6, on the outside of the loop and raised slightly from the road, is the pick of the loop. Score this site and you can set your tent back into a secluded grove of trees, with terrific mountain views to the east and west. B8 has a great spot for a tent, perfect morning sun, and a mix of quaking aspens and conifers. But although this is a beautiful site, it isn't as private as some of the others.

Loop C, which actually sits below Loop B, affords views of Quake Lake and the mountains to the south. As you drop into Loop C, you'll encounter a delightful aspen grove, and Quake Lake sits just below, full of rainbows, browns, and cutthroats using the dead trees, still standing from 1959, for cover. An interesting hogback ridge runs up the mountainside that dominates the landscape in front of you. Mountain bluebells and lupines provide splashes of color.

A few prime sites exist on Loop C. Site C13 sits back from the road just a bit and offers a picturesque open spot for tents. Site C20 puts you on the outside of the loop, providing a nice backdrop of the mountains and plenty of flat space to set up a tent. Site C18 is on the outside of the loop; back your car in, and you will block your neighbor's view of your picnic table while you enjoy your morning tea or coffee and soak in the terrific mountain views.

A walk down to the lake may provide a chance sighting of a moose. During busy months, animals are more likely to seek cover away from the campground.

Beaver Creek Campground

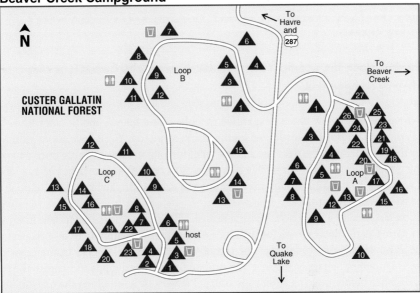

GETTING THERE

From West Yellowstone, take US 191 north for 8 miles to Hebgen Lake Road (US 287). Turn left and go west for 16 miles to the campground.

GPS COORDINATES: N44° 51.683' W111° 22.367'

29

⛺ Falls Creek Campground

Beauty: ★★★★ / Privacy: ★★★★★ / Quiet: ★★★★★ / Spaciousness: ★★★★★ / Security: ★★★★ / Cleanliness: ★★★★★

Situated along the scenic Main Boulder River, Falls Creek is a rare tent-only campground.

The drive to Falls Creek bisects expansive ranchland and follows the Boulder River as it winds through an isolated section of south-central Montana. You'll have plenty of time to enjoy the mountains in the distance and the wildlife along the way, because once you come to the gravel road, the only survivable speed is a slow one. Along the way, you can stop in McLeod at Holly's Road Kill Cafe for something to eat and drink and a game of pool, and some friendly conversation.

A bit farther down the road is Natural Bridge, where a spectacular waterfall show peaks every spring as the natural rock formations and river come together here in a magical way. Some days, the river cascades over the top of the rocks in a tumbling, frothing, swirling mass. On others, when the water level has dropped, the water disappears beneath the rocks for a distance before pouring from gaps situated at various levels along the canyon. Interpretive signs help visitors understand the geology of the area, and paved trails and overlooks make access easy. Extreme care should be taken, since there are no guardrails along the edge of some trail sections. The easiest hike in the area (but still a challenge) is an 11-mile out-and-back from here to Green Mountain and the East Boulder Campground.

Not much farther down the road is your goal: Falls Creek—a rare find with virtually everything a car camper could ask for, from its setting along the scenic Boulder River to its tents-only design. The river provides a world-class trout habitat and lives up to its name with behemoth boulders forcing the flow into a whitewater frenzy.

Sites here are all walk-in; they line the river's edge with views of the cliffs on the opposite shore, and the walk to your site is less than 100 yards. Site 2 is closest to the water, located on a bend in the river and set off from the others, but sites 1 and 3 overlook it since it lies between them and the river. Site 1 is private, and the setting is good, but it is closer to the parking area and a little farther (maybe 30 yards) from the water. Sites 3 and 4 are fairly close to one another, and although there are plenty of firs and cottonwoods between them, the shade prevents much understory privacy. All sites are roomy, and you can easily set up camp without being on top of your neighbor. If you want privacy, site 8 is totally hidden. The downside is that it isn't on the water, and the surrounding trees and brush block most

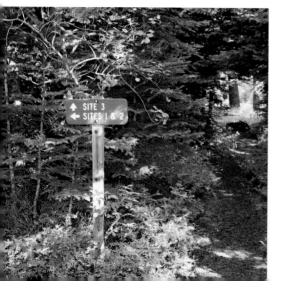

Campers at Falls Creek Campground enjoy wooded campsites next to the Boulder River.

KEY INFORMATION

ADDRESS: MT 298, Big Timber, MT 59011

CONTACT: 406-222-1892, www.fs.usda.gov
/custergallatin

OPERATED BY: Custer Gallatin National
Forest, Yellowstone Ranger District

OPEN: Year-round when accessible; water
available late May–September

SITES: 8 (walk-in)

EACH SITE: Picnic table, fire ring

ASSIGNMENT: First come, first served;
no reservations

REGISTRATION: None

FACILITIES: Hand-pump well, vault toilets

PARKING: A short walk from each campsite

FEE: Free

ELEVATION: 5,200'

RESTRICTIONS:

Pets: On leash only

Fires: In fire rings only

Alcohol: Permitted

Vehicles: No RVs or trailers

Other: 16-day stay limit; bear-country
food storage restrictions; pack in,
pack out

of the river view. At this end of the campground, site 7 offers the best combination of privacy, proximity to water, and scenic view. Much of the land in this area is privately owned, including property along the river. The water itself is public, as are some portions of the riverbank, but take time to familiarize yourself with the state's stream-access regulations to avoid trespassing.

If this picture-perfect campground is full—a possibility if you don't arrive early on weekends and holidays—you'll find several other developed campgrounds as you continue south. In 2.4 miles you come to Big Beaver Campground. A half mile farther is

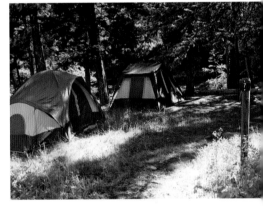

Falls Creek Campground is a family-friendly tent-only option.

the more secluded Aspen Campground, and two tent-only sites nestle along the river at Chippy Park, 4.5 miles south of Falls Creek.

Hiking in this area is not for the weak of heart (or legs). The scenery and wildlife are spectacular, but so are the elevation gains. Below Two-Mile Bridge on the west side of the road is the trailhead for Great Falls Creek Trail #18, a hike up several switchbacks to 10,604-foot West Boulder Plateau in the Absaroka-Beartooth Wilderness. It's an extremely strenuous 9 miles to the plateau, making this more than a day hike for all but the heartiest hikers. You could, however, hike partway out and back: you'll still be in the wilderness, and it's all downhill coming home.

Another mile down the road on the east side is Graham Creek Trail #117, which runs between Chrome Mountain and Contact Mountain on the way to the East Boulder Plateau. This is another steep (4,300'-elevation-gain) hike that isn't technically in the wilderness, but you won't be able to tell by the scenery. Off the west side of the road before the entrance to Falls Creek is Grouse Creek Trail #14, which winds 7 miles to West Boulder Campground.

Falls Creek Campground

GETTING THERE

From Big Timber, take MT 298 south for 30 miles to the campground. (Don't take the turn-off to East Boulder Road.)

GPS COORDINATES: N45° 29.416' W110° 13.086'

30

Greenough Lake Campground

Beauty: ★★★★★ / Privacy: ★★★★ / Quiet: ★★★★ / Spaciousness: ★★★★ / Security: ★★★★ /
Cleanliness: ★★★★★

This canyon campground sits in a thick pine-and-fir forest along Rock Creek at the foot of Beartooth Pass.

Set amid spectacular forests and mountain scenery, the narrow Red Lodge Valley has a history of coal mining, colorful and eccentric Old West characters, outdoor recreation, and rodeo royalty. Yes, rodeo royalty. This is the valley where Ben Greenough led pack trains through the steep mountains and across the lofty plateaus of the Beartooths for years, and where his eight children grew up riding horses. Five of them participated in rodeos: Turk was named King of the Bronc Riders in 1935, and Alice and Marge rode both bulls and bucking broncos to win a wealth of championships around the world.

The Greenoughs helped bring organized rodeo to Red Lodge and helped build an arena in 1929 for locals who had been competing at the railroad stockyards since before the turn of the century. Another local hero, Bill Linderman, added more titles to the town's history, even winning the title of "World All-Around Champion" three times. His brother Bud won a world championship as well, and in their honor the Red Lodge rodeo was renamed "Home of Champions Rodeo." Today the tradition continues, with brothers Quinn, Trey, and Turk Greenough—Alice Greenough's great-great-nephews—making their mark on the sport.

Willie Nelson was giving a concert at the rodeo grounds in August 2000 when a motorcycle crash ignited a wildfire that spread over 2,000 acres in a few hours. Naming forest fires is a function of the local ranger district, and the name must be distinctive enough to allow differentiation between it and past or future fires. This one was named Willie, thus making Nelson the only professional entertainer to have a forest fire named after him—a dubious honor, don't you think?

A few miles south of the fire area are Rock Creek Road and the turnoff for Greenough Lake, a canyon campground that is set in a thick pine-and-fir forest along Rock Creek at the foot of Beartooth Pass. The sites along the creek are the best, with 1, 2, and 3 all providing privacy and plenty of room. Of the trio, site 3 is the best, with the most understory buffering the view of the loop road. Creekside sites 5 and 7 are large and private; they are

Headwaters of Rock Creek

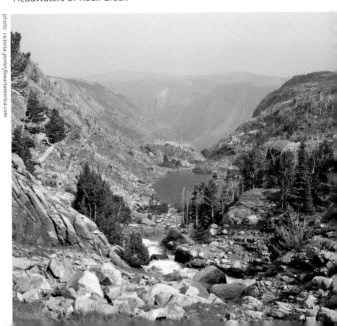

photo: victoria-porter/fineartamerica.com

ADDRESS: Main Fork Road (Forest Road 2421), Red Lodge, MT 59068

CONTACT: 406-446-2103, www.fs.usda.gov /custergallatin; reservations: 877-444-6777, recreation.gov

OPERATED BY: Custer Gallatin National Forest, Beartooth Ranger District

OPEN: May–September

SITES: 18

EACH SITE: Picnic table, fire ring

ASSIGNMENT: First come, first served and by reservation

REGISTRATION: On-site self-registration

FACILITIES: Hand-pump well, vault toilets

PARKING: At campsites

FEE: $17, $9/additional vehicle

ELEVATION: 7,300'

RESTRICTIONS:

Pets: On leash only

Fires: In fire rings only

Alcohol: Permitted

Vehicles: 32-foot length limit

Other: 16-day stay limit; bear-country food storage restrictions

also among the few sites you can't reserve. Site 13 is the most unusual, with a huge boulder that just begs to be climbed.

Although deer and elk are the most plentiful, moose frequently visit the area, and at least a few bears will appear throughout the summer. A short trail leads from the campground to Greenough Lake. This small lake, named for the local rodeo dynasty, is stocked with rainbow trout, and at less than 10 feet deep, it's popular for family fishing outings during which kids frequently land good-sized keepers.

Across a bridge and directly on the opposite bank of Rock Creek is Limber Pine Campground, where you can reserve the best sites—site 9 on a bluff above the creek and site 8 down below for views of the creek and more privacy.

The trailhead for Glacier Lake Trail #3 is 8 miles down the gravel road past Limber Pine. High-clearance 4x4 vehicles are recommended to drive this rocky, primitive road to the trailhead. (Pro-tip from a ranger: before you start your hike, sprinkle moth crystals or salt

The best sites at Greenough Lake Campground are located next to Rock Creek.

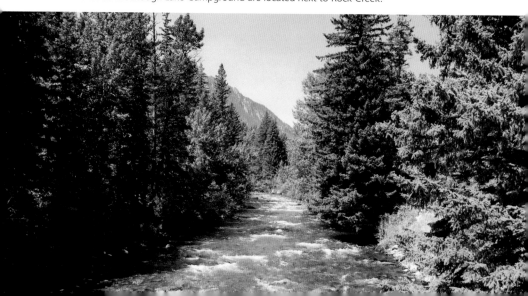

around your vehicle to ward off marmots, which are known to snack on radiator hoses and car wiring and can cause extensive vehicle damage.) This trail to the Rock Creek headwaters begins at about 8,600 feet and climbs steeply along Moon Creek for 1.7 miles and ending on a ridge above the tree line before it drops down to the bowl where the lake nestles at 9,700 feet on the Montana–Wyoming border. Trails lead to several other lakes in this basin, but the fishing here and in adjacent Little Glacier Lake generally yields larger cutthroat and brook trout. The wind picks up in the afternoon, and short but severe storms can roll in suddenly, bringing rain, hail, and even snow.

Rock Creek also provides sections of Class III and IV whitewater, with a put-in at Lake Fork Creek, 11 miles south of Red Lodge. Lower Lake Fork Trail #1 into the Absaroka-Beartooth Wilderness is an easy-to-moderate 2.9-mile out-and-back hike through the forest alongside the creek's whitewater and waterfalls. The trail skirts Black Pyramid Mountain and is an excellent place to see moose.

While hiking, you may see what looks like pink snow. No, you're not seeing things—the snow really is pink, particularly in late summer, and is often called watermelon snow. The color is due to an algae (*Chlamydomonas nivalis*) that turns red as it thrives in the warm summer sun. You may find that hiking through these snowfields discolors your boot soles, socks, and pant cuffs, but don't worry; it's only temporary.

Greenough Lake Campground

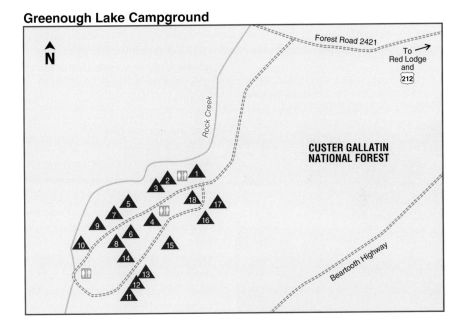

GETTING THERE

From Red Lodge, take US 212 southwest for 12 miles to Forest Road 2421. Turn right and go 1 mile southwest to the campground.

GPS COORDINATES: N45° 3.367' W109° 24.767'

31

Halfmoon Campground

Beauty: ★★★★★ / Privacy: ★★★★★ / Quiet: ★★★★★ / Spaciousness: ★★★★★ / Security: ★★★★ / Cleanliness: ★★★★

Big Timber and Crazy Peaks loom to the southwest, and 2,000-foot rock-canyon walls rise on either side of the campground.

The drive into Halfmoon Campground is rocky and slow, but the scenery is what tourists expect to see in Montana: a spectacular mountain range bursting from a valley floor carpeted with ranchland and speckled with cows grazing between the sagebrush. One of the state's island ranges, the Crazy Mountains rise stunningly out of nowhere and confirm for those driving west on I-90 that, yes indeed, they have finally made it to the Rocky Mountains.

Called *Awaxaawippiia* by the Crow, the Crazy Mountains are where Chief Plenty Coups received his leadership vision, and the range remains a sacred, spiritual place for the tribe. As for how the mountains were named, a variety of stories exist, and everyone has their favorite. Be sure to ask locals for their version.

The Crazy Mountains are not sprawling but compact, extending only about 25 miles; what they lack in breadth, however, they make up for in height, with two dozen peaks towering above 10,000 feet. On the western flank is Grasshopper Glacier, a lingering remnant of the glaciers that, like a sculptor's chisel, carved these mountains by etching away mud and stone. Created some 50 million years earlier, the glacier appeared when magma rose from deep within the earth's core to the muddy ocean floor and solidified into igneous rock.

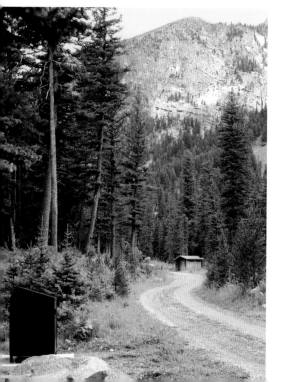

The Crazy Mountains provide a stunning backdrop to camping at Halfmoon Campground.

Much of the land in this area falls under so-called checkerboard ownership, meaning that if you look at an ownership map of the area, the mix of public and private land resembles a checkerboard. Because the approach to Halfmoon passes through private property, respecting private land during your visit is not only important but also simply the right thing to do. When you come to a gate on the campground entrance road, please be sure to close it behind you.

This is a busy place on holidays and weekends, and it's not hard to understand why. Your first thought when you arrive at Halfmoon may be much like ours—we don't need to go anywhere else; this is perfection. The setting is amazingly, spectacularly, dramatically

ADDRESS: Big Timber Canyon Road,
Big Timber, MT 59011

CONTACT: 406-222-1892, www.fs.usda.gov
/custergallatin

OPERATED BY: Custer Gallatin National
Forest, Yellowstone Ranger District

OPEN: Memorial Day–September,
weather permitting

SITES: 12

EACH SITE: Picnic table, fire grate

ASSIGNMENT: First come, first served;
no reservations

REGISTRATION: On-site self-registration

FACILITIES: Hand-pump well, vault toilets

PARKING: At campsites

FEE: $5

ELEVATION: 6,500'

RESTRICTIONS:

Pets: On leash only

Fires: In fire rings only

Alcohol: Permitted

Vehicles: 32-foot length limit

Other: 16-day stay limit; bear-country
food storage restrictions; pack in,
pack out

breathtaking—Big Timber Peak (10,795')
and Crazy Peak (11,214') loom to the southwest, and 2,000-foot rock-canyon walls rise
on either side of the campground. Stubby
Douglas-firs are evidence of the short
growing season, but they're more than
large enough to provide effective shade and
privacy screening. Moss-covered boulders
are a subtle indication that melting winter
snows last well into summer.

Each of the dozen sites here is somewhat secluded. You're still going to see
other people, but each site has plenty of
space for a tent and is outfitted with the
standard table and fire ring. Everything
is in place for a relaxing evening spent

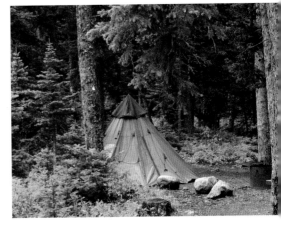

A typical campsite at Halfmoon

enjoying dinner and scanning the cliffs with binoculars to spot mountain goats clinging to
the edges.

Adjacent to the campground is Big Timber Creek Trail #119, where you can take a very
short hike to the lower portion of Big Timber Falls (also known as Halfmoon Falls) or continue less than 0.5 miles to the upper falls. Three miles down Trail 119, you'll run into Blue
Lake Trail #118, a 1.5-mile spur to Blue Lake, where the fishing is good and the setting for a
picnic is superb. A few miles past the Blue Lake Spur, you'll come to Conical Peak.

Even though the trails can get busy on weekends, birds are easy to spot, with eagles and
hawks in the sky and an occasional wild turkey rattling the shrubs. Black bears, deer, mountain lions, elk, and mountain goats make hiking an observation adventure. Wildflowers are
abundant in some sections and bloom later than those at lower elevations. Because much
of the land here is privately owned and is designated as such, please stay on the trails and be
respectful of the property and its owners.

Yes, it can snow any time of year at Halfmoon, but we're betting that once you're here, it will be hard to tear yourself away.

Halfmoon Campground

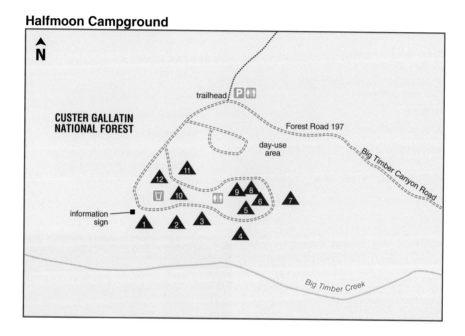

GETTING THERE

From Big Timber, take US 191 north for 11 miles to Big Timber Canyon Road (Wormser Loop Road). Turn left and go 15 miles west to the campground.

GPS COORDINATES: N46° 2.463' W110° 14.288'

32

Hood Creek Campground

Beauty: ★★★★★ / Privacy: ★★★★ / Quiet: ★★★ / Spaciousness: ★★★★★ / Security: ★★★★ /
Cleanliness: ★★★★

Hood Creek is lakeside surrounded by mountains, wildflower meadows, and waterfalls.

Built in the 1940s to provide water for area farms and ranches, Hyalite Reservoir is the anchor for a recreation area attracting hikers, campers, anglers, and those just seeking a little time to relax outdoors. Due to its close proximity to Bozeman, it's a prime recreation destination for locals and Montana State University students, so reservations are recommended.

You'll find several U.S. Forest Service campgrounds here, but Hood Creek is our choice for tenters. While there are more RVs nowadays than there used to be, you can still find privacy here; again, though, reserving ahead is advisable if you want a prime site.

Hood Creek is spread in a narrow band along the reservoir, providing plenty of room between sites as well as a lot of space within the sites themselves. Reservations are accepted for all of the sites here. Site 28 is a group site and sites 21–23 are day-use picnic sites located at the boat ramp.

The reservoir's setting is pretty remarkable for an artificial body of water. Surrounded by mountains, wildflower meadows, and waterfalls, this area draws a variety of wildlife and birds. There is a no-wake policy on the 1.25-mile-long lake, where canoes and sailboats are plentiful, along with cutthroat trout and arctic grayling. The no-wake policy is enforced and helps keep noise down.

The entire canyon is a paradise for hikers, with trails for all skill and stamina levels around every bend. The turnoff for History Rock Trail #424 is on the west side of the road, 1 mile before the reservoir. This fairly steep 3.5-mile trail leads to an outcropping carved with historic graffiti left by early settlers. Unfortunately, more recent (and careless) visitors often leave their marks as well. The trail continues from here for 3 miles to Cottonwood Creek and unless you're prepared to spend the night on the trail, this will be the turnaround point. The trailhead for Blackmore Trail #423 is at the Blackmore Picnic Area before the reservoir bridge. This trail leads to the peak of Mount Blackmore (10,154').

You can hike to Hyalite Peak from the trailhead about 2 miles past Hood

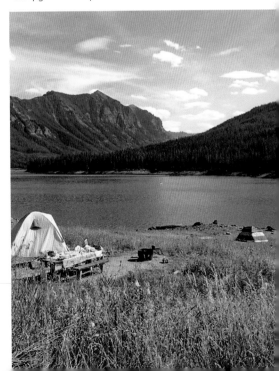

Situated on the shoreline of a stunning reservoir surrounded by magnificent mountains, Hood Creek Campground is a prime recreational destination.

KEY INFORMATION

ADDRESS: Hyalite Canyon Road, Bozeman, MT 59718

CONTACT: 406-522-2520, www.fs.usda.gov/custergallatin; reservations: 877-444-6777, recreation.gov

OPERATED BY: Yellowstone Country Campgrounds

OPEN: Mid-May–October, weather permitting (no drinking water past mid-September)

SITES: 25 standard sites plus 1 group site

EACH SITE: Picnic table, fire ring

ASSIGNMENT: First come, first served and by reservation

REGISTRATION: On-site self-registration

FACILITIES: Hand-pump well, vault toilets, boat ramp, picnic area, firewood for sale

PARKING: At campsites

FEE: $15, $7/additional vehicle

ELEVATION: 6,700'

RESTRICTIONS:

Pets: On leash only

Fires: In fire rings only

Alcohol: Permitted

Vehicles: Variable length limits, maximum 47 feet

Other: 16-day stay limit; bear-country food storage restrictions; pack in, pack out

Creek. The view from the peak is spectacular, as are the 11 waterfalls along the way. On this 14-mile out-and-back hike, the first half of the trail climbs so gently you probably won't notice you're climbing, although there are a few steep sections. Then the grade gets steeper, and you'll encounter a dozen or so switchbacks. Hyalite Lake sits in a wide, deep basin just past the 5-mile mark; hike the last 2 miles to the top of Hyalite Peak (10,299'). Overall, the elevation gain is about 3,300 feet, taking you to a height where snow usually hangs around until July and often returns by Labor Day.

Recreation, scenery, wildlife—there's something for everybody at Hood Creek Campground.

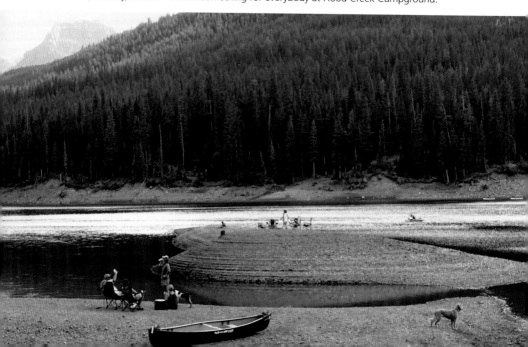

The trailhead for Palisade Falls National Recreation Trail is located past Hood Creek and to the left at the Y. This paved 0.6-mile trail snakes through a forest of pine, fir, and spruce to the 98-foot falls.

The trailhead for East Fork Hyalite Trail #434 is about 1 mile farther down East Fork Road. This 11-mile out-and-back trail follows the East Fork of Hyalite Creek, a fast-running haven for cutthroat and brook trout and grayling. The climb is gradual for the first few miles with only one steep section as it moves through the forested creek bottoms. Once you pass Horsetail Falls, the grade increases, as does the expansiveness of the views. You'll face a dozen switchbacks before you get to Emerald and Heather Lakes, but this isn't a difficult hike.

In this region you'll find mountainsides dropping steeply down to lakeshores and a wealth of rocky cliffs. On any of these trails you'll be greeted by a wildflower display that evolves all summer, and wildlife viewing is generally good, especially if you're looking for elk, deer, or mountain goats.

Hood Creek Campground

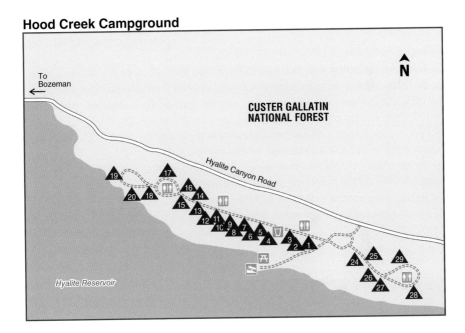

GETTING THERE

From Bozeman, take 19th Street south for 7 miles to Hyalite Canyon Road. Turn left and continue south for 10 miles (crossing over the bridge at the reservoir) to the campground.

GPS COORDINATES: N45° 29.100' W110° 58.067'

33

⛺ Potosi Campground

Beauty: ★★★★★ / Privacy: ★★★ / Quiet: ★★★★ / Spaciousness: ★★★ / Security: ★★★★ /
Cleanliness: ★★★★

You'll have great trail access at this basic campground in a spectacular setting.

Visitors to this section of Montana's Tobacco Root Range can take advantage of several hiking trails leading to pristine lakes, set beneath rugged cliffs that provide spectacular homes to mountain goat herds throughout the summer. The range is not the highest in the state, but it is steep, and pitches of over 45 degrees are not uncommon. The not-quite-a-ghost-town of Pony is perched in a narrow opening and is a pleasant stop before heading deeper into the mountains. A few reminders of the area's short-lived silver-mining history are scattered along the drive to the campground, but they pale in comparison to the peaceful scenery that just keeps on getting better.

A big plus is the lure of the hot springs. A larger springs is on private property, but the public upper springs can be reached from the campground trailhead on the east side of the creek. Follow the easy first mile of Forest Service Trail #308 along South Willow Creek, and when the creek widens, start looking along the creekbed for the log fencing enclosing the hot springs. Climb through the fencing to access the springs. Both are small, and a group of six will fill them to capacity.

Access to the campground can be confusing, as it sits astride South Willow Creek, with five sites on the west bank and the rest on the east bank; watch for a post with a tent sign at the access roads. A thick forest envelops these compact sites, and even though sites on the west bank are on the creek, sites on the other loop are more private and almost as close to the water. Site 8, on the east loop, is the most spacious and offers the most seclusion; a small stream runs behind it and site 7. If all of the sites are filled, several dispersed sites are a good option, since they are still close to the water pump and outhouses.

South Willow Creek channels through the middle of Potosi Campground.

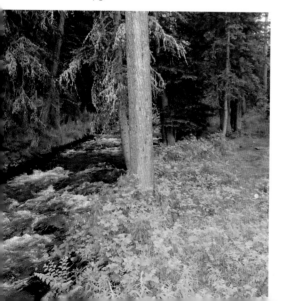

Fishing in the creek provides lucky anglers with rainbow, brown, brook, and cutthroat trout, while waders just enjoy the clear, cool water that is a refreshing contrast to the nearby hot springs.

This is a popular place for locals, and you'll encounter a lot of motorized traffic on some trails, especially on the weekends. For those who have ATVs or motorbikes, this is an ideal location. Mountain bikers and hikers shouldn't necessarily shy away, however, since many trails have restrictions that help everyone share this corner of the

Tobacco Root Range. Wildlife viewing is good for mule deer, elk, moose, and black bears.

Potosi Trail #303 heads west from where the road splits between the campground loops and is solid switchbacks for the first mile to the ridge overlooking the creek that weaves through the campground. The trail runs along the ridge and then climbs another mile before intersecting with primitive Rock Creek Trail #304. Past the intersection, it climbs sharply to another ridge and the Albro Lake and North Willow Creek trail systems. Follow Trail #304 down to South Willow Creek Road, and you'll be about a mile from the campground. This is a strenuous but manageable 6-mile hike or mountain bike loop.

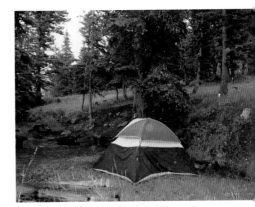

Campsites here are simple yet roomy.

Two miles west of Pony is the trailhead for North Willow Creek Trail #301. This trail follows the north side of the creek for 3 miles and then crosses to the south side for the final 2-mile climb to Hollowtop Lake. The last section is rocky, but not too steep. ATVs are allowed only on the first mile of this trail, and motorcycles are prohibited off the trail and around the lake. Another option after the first mile is to take the turnoff to Albro Lake Trail #333, a 5-mile hike to an alpine lake. The trail climbs through mountain meadows with valley views before dropping to the bowl surrounding the lake.

Bell Lake Trail #305 follows the north side of the creek, and for the first 2.5 miles, climbs slowly to a gate where only motorcycles, people, and horses can continue the last mile, a tough climb to the lake. It's hard to believe that at one time, vehicles used this same route to get to Bell Lake.

Potosi Campground

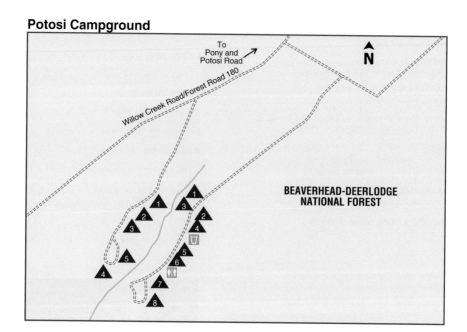

GETTING THERE

From Harrison, take MT 283 west for 6.5 miles to Pony. Turn left on Potosi Road and, after about 3 miles, turn right on South Willow Creek Road. Continue about 8 miles to a left turnoff for the east campground loop. Or drive another 0.2 miles on South Willow Creek Road to the west-loop turnoff, and continue to the campground.

GPS COORDINATES: N45° 34.331' W111° 54.809'

34

Sheridan Campground

Beauty: ★★★★ / Privacy: ★★★★ / Quiet: ★★★★ / Spaciousness: ★★★★★ / Security: ★★★★★ /
Cleanliness: ★★★★

Rock Creek rushes along the western edge of this campground.

Red Lodge is the gateway to one of the most scenic drives in the United States. The 70-mile-long Beartooth Highway, a National Scenic Byway and an All-American Road, ascends out of Red Lodge through Rock Creek Canyon, serving up spectacular views as it winds to Cooke City and then into Yellowstone National Park. Built between 1931 and 1936 at a cost of $2.5 million, this spectacular highway allows anyone with the nerve to experience what was once only visible to those on foot or horseback: profuse wildflower carpets and a high alpine environment at elevations above 10,000 feet. The sharp switchbacks, unpredictable weather, and remarkable views make each trip on the Beartooth an adventure.

With dramatic, forested peaks surrounding you, it's hard to believe this was once a hotbed of mining activity. Cooke City was home to the New World Mining District, from where gold and silver ore were transported to Red Lodge and beyond. But it was the rich coal beds east of Red Lodge that gave rise to the towns of Washoe and Bearcreek, where mines thrived in the first half of the 20th century, and the valley population peaked at more than 7,000. The mines survived the Depression but were devastated in 1943 when 74 miners died in an explosion at the Smith Mine. This was the state's worst mining disaster and the beginning of the end for large-scale mining in the area.

Six miles south of Red Lodge is Sheridan, the first of several U.S. Forest Service campgrounds along the beginning of the Beartooth Highway. A great spot to set up base camp

Pig racing at the Bear Creek Saloon

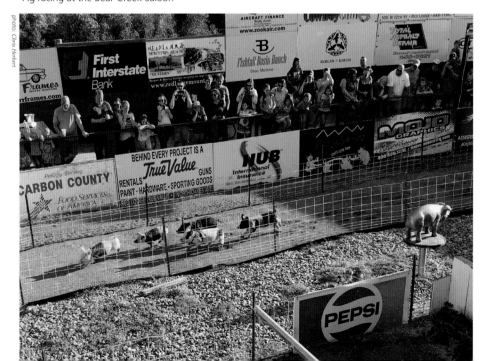

photo: *Chris Herbert*

KEY INFORMATION

ADDRESS: East Side Road, Red Lodge, MT 59068

CONTACT: 406-446-2103, www.fs.usda.gov /custergallatin; reservations: 877-444-6777, recreation.gov

OPERATED BY: Custer Gallatin National Forest, Beartooth Ranger District

OPEN: Memorial Day weekend–Labor Day

SITES: 9

EACH SITE: Picnic table, fire rings

ASSIGNMENT: First come, first served or by reservation

REGISTRATION: Self-registration online

FACILITIES: Hand-pump water, vault toilets

PARKING: At campsites

FEE: $16, $9/additional vehicle

ELEVATION: 6,300'

RESTRICTIONS:

Pets: On leash only

Fires: In fire rings only

Alcohol: Permitted

Vehicles: 30-foot length limit

Other: 16-day stay limit; bear-country food storage restrictions

for a few days of exploring this awe-inspiring piece of Montana, Sheridan is small, consisting of just nine campsites. Rock Creek rushes along the western edge of the campground, masking any roadway noise and providing great opportunities for fishing or cooling off in the summer sun. Try to score site 8 or 9 if you can. They're the largest sites and have plenty of tent space, dynamite 360-degree views, sun, shade, and access to the creek. Large and shady site 7 is another good pick, with level tent space and beautiful views of the surrounding area. The campground's access to the creek is between sites 8 and 9, but there's enough room that it isn't intrusive. Sheridan is also a good place for a group, since sites 1 and 2 can be reserved together.

Just south of Red Lodge is West Fork Road (Forest Road 2071) and access to Basin Lakes National Recreation Trail #6. This is moderate 4.8-mile hike along the West Fork Rock Creek leads to a pair of high-mountain lakes where the biggest challenges are the last steep mile and how long to spend fishing. On the way to Basin Lakes Trail, you'll see plenty of mountain bikers on West Fork Road and the old logging roads that spoke off into the steep and rugged terrain.

Also off US 212 is the Meeteetse Trail, a 19-mile route recommended for 4x4 and high-clearance vehicles as it travels over undulating hills that wind through a mix of sagebrush-filled flats and lush river bottoms. Sightings of antelope, deer, and moose are frequent, with hawks and golden eagles plentiful as well. The Face of the Mountain trailhead and Trail #7 are located on the road 3 miles west of Red Lodge.

Hiking trails generally lead into the Absaroka-Beartooth Wilderness and can be used for day hikes as well as longer backpacking trips. Elevation gains and switchbacks are the norm, and knowing your limits both in terms of time and stamina are important. The ranger-district office in Red Lodge is an important stop for trail maps and current information.

While you're in town, check out Yellowstone Wildlife Sanctuary, a wildlife rehabilitation center in Coal Miner's Park, and visit the Carbon County Museum, where you can learn about folks like Calamity Jane, Liver Eating Johnson, Buffalo Bill, John Colter, and Jim Bridger, along with the rainbow of ethnic groups that have called Red Lodge home.

For one of the most unique experiences in the state, stop at the Bear Creek Saloon and Steakhouse Thursday–Sunday between Memorial Day and Labor Day to place your bets during the pig races. It's hard to tell who's having more fun, the people or the pigs, but area students are the ultimate winners: the proceeds fund several college scholarships.

Sheridan Campground

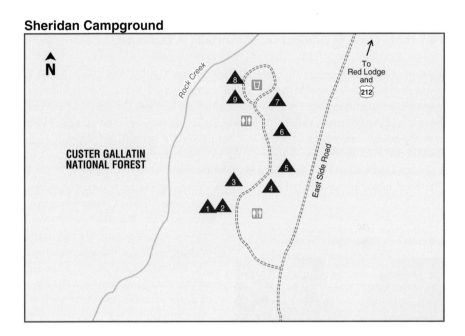

GETTING THERE

From Red Lodge, take US 212 south for 6 miles to East Side Road. Turn left and go 2 miles south to the campground.

GPS COORDINATES: N45° 5.954' W109° 18.446'

35

Spire Rock Campground

Beauty: ★★★★ / Privacy: ★★★★ / Quiet: ★★★★ / Spaciousness: ★★★★ / Security: ★★★★ /
Cleanliness: ★★★★

At the doorstep of activities and attractions where you can also have a great tent-camping experience, essentially in seclusion.

By the time you turn off scenic Highway 191 onto Storm Castle Creek Road (Forest Road 132), you may be wondering whether great tent camping awaits you. The turnoff comes a little more than 10 minutes after you enter Gallatin Canyon from the north, where you left the busyness of the Bozeman Valley. The thickening spruce-and-fir forest along the Gallatin River is appealing—but what's with the U.S. Forest Service helipad and riverside pullouts and, where the road bends away from the river to follow Storm Castle Creek, a parking lot with two trailheads receiving a fair share of attention?

The good news: you've entered a picturesque canyon where recreational activities are numerous. The bad news: there isn't any activity. Your campsite is located well beyond the river pullouts and trailhead parking lot, all of which will empty by day's end as tired fun seekers head home. You, on the other hand, remain at the doorstep of all the activities and attractions, where you can also have a great tent camping experience, essentially in seclusion.

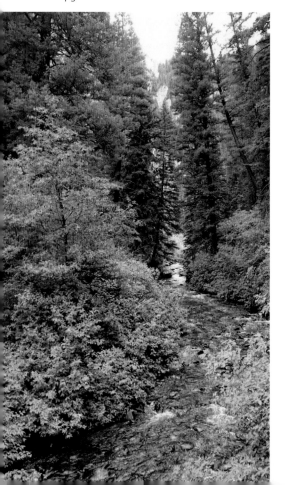

Storm Castle Creek and forest buffer Spire Rock Campground from Storm Castle Creek Road.

So relax and keep your focus on the road to the campground entrance, just a mile beyond the trailheads and parking lot. You enter the campground by taking a right at the campground sign. Immediately, once over the creek on a bridge, you'll find 20 campsites sitting on both sides of the road, which runs parallel to the creek. The campground road is not a loop but a thru-route to the exit on the east, which is always nice: a one-way road reduces traffic from campers coming and going.

The setting is tranquil, with the pleasant sound of Storm Castle Creek punctuating the background. If you like the gentle sound of a creek, choose a campsite next to the creek, although you can hear the creek from all sites. The campsites are suitable for tents, and most offer plenty of space between one another.

KEY INFORMATION

ADDRESS: Storm Castle Creek Road
(Forest Road 132), Bozeman, MT 59718

CONTACT: 406-522-2520, www.fs.usda.gov
/custergallatin; reservations: 877-444-
6777, recreation.gov

OPERATED BY: Yellowstone Country
Campgrounds

OPEN: May–September

SITES: 20

EACH SITE: Picnic table, fire ring

ASSIGNMENT: First come, first served;
or online at recreation.gov

REGISTRATION: On-site self-registration

FACILITIES: Vault toilets but no
drinking water

PARKING: At campsites

FEE: $11, $7/additional vehicle

ELEVATION: 5,600'

RESTRICTIONS:

Pets: On leash only

Fires: In fire rings only

Alcohol: Permitted

Vehicles: 30-foot length limit,
2 vehicles/site

Other: 16-day stay limit; firewood;
bear-country food storage restrictions

The campground is situated on the north side of Garnet Mountain, which casts a cool shadow on the campground for a good portion of the day, which is a bonus during the warmer summer months. Garnet Mountain has a fire lookout tower at its 8,245-foot summit (the lookout sleeps four and can be reserved for overnight stays at recreation.gov). Accessed at the south side of the Storm Castle trailhead, at the parking lot you passed, the 3.5-mile hike to the summit on Garnet Mountain Trail #85 gains impressive panoramic views of surrounding mountains, highlighted by the Spanish Peaks to the west and the Gallatin River Valley below, also to the west. Hyalite Ridge is viewed to the east and the Gallatin Range to the east and south.

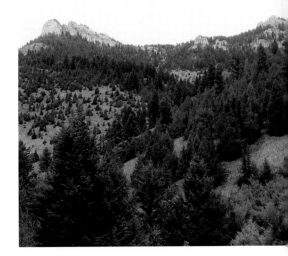

Storm Castle Peak looms to the northwest of Spire Rock. Its summit can be reached by hiking a moderately steep trail.

The Storm Castle Trail is named for the 7,165-foot tower looming over the parking lot to the north. The popular hike up the south-facing slope to the summit of Storm Castle Peak is on a moderately steep trail, but the 4.7-mile round-trip hike is worth it for the views and opportunity to see wildlife.

The vehicle pullouts next to the Gallatin River along Storm Castle Creek Road are frequented daily by anglers seeking the scrappy rainbow and brown trout lurking below. If you're also intent on tapping into the action, you can avoid the roadside stretch by hiking up the Garnet Mountain Trail for a short distance until you arrive at a split in the trail. Take the trail to the right and hike it to a sweet spot at the river.

Upstream, the Gallatin River is very popular for independent and guided floating, and the House Rock and Mad Mile sections are particularly popular for the paddling community that enjoys Class III rapids or harder thrills. The section accessed below these more challenging runs is easily scouted and favored by less-skilled floaters. It can be accessed at numerous points along Highway 191, with a good takeout upstream but near Storm Castle Creek Road.

Spire Rock Campground

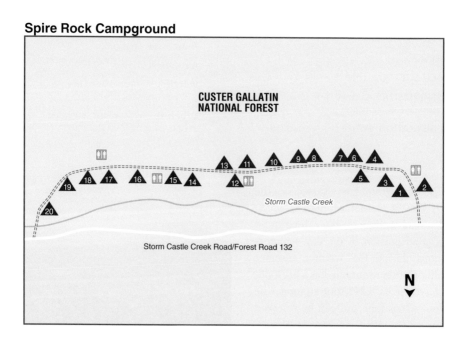

GETTING THERE

From Four Corners, travel south for 19 miles on MT 191 to Storm Castle Creek Road (FR 132). Turn left, cross a single-lane bridge, and travel a gravel road 3 miles to the campground.

GPS COORDINATES: N45° 26.483' W111° 12.383'

36

Swan Creek Campground

Beauty: ★★★★ / Privacy: ★★★★ / Quiet: ★★★★ / Spaciousness: ★★★★ / Security: ★★★★ / Cleanliness: ★★★★

This is a small, densely forested campground in Gallatin Canyon.

Tucked between the Madison and Gallatin Ranges, US 191 follows the spectacular narrow canyon that winds alongside the Gallatin River from Bozeman to the west entrance of Yellowstone National Park. Driving this route is a study in contrasts, from the historic but closed Gallatin Gateway Hotel, built by the Milwaukee Road in the 1920s, to the sprawling development of the town and ski resort of Big Sky.

Along the way are vast sections of unspoiled scenery sprinkled with guest ranches and private cabins. It's tough to take it all in when you're behind the wheel. Drivers must be vigilant of the heavy truck traffic, narrow winding roadway, and blind corners. Truckers may get impatient (since there aren't any passing zones), but take your time anyway. If cars are backed up behind you, stop in one of the pullout spots and let them pass. Remember, you're on vacation. Besides, while you're stopped you can get out of the car and explore the riverbank. There's a good chance you'll see floating parties bobbing by as they take on the river's challenging Class II, III, and IV whitewater. Guided trips are prevalent due to the technical difficulty, and outfitters are available in Big Sky and Bozeman.

Taking some time to fish on this blue-ribbon trout stream is always an excellent choice. Swan Creek offers enough mountain whitefish and rainbow, brown, cutthroat, and brook trout to challenge and delight any angler.

Swan Creek is on the east side of the highway, but the turnoff sign for Forest Road 481 doesn't give you much warning. Keep an eye on your odometer and the mileage markers, and you'll be fine. If you do miss the turn, there are plenty of places to turn around and backtrack. Swan Creek sits a mile off the highway, which makes it the quietest option among the five campgrounds along the canyon. But it is a popular place and nine of the sites here can be reserved. You should take advantage of that option if possible, as campsites fill up quickly by Friday afternoon.

Swan Creek is a small, densely forested campground with sites split into two small sections about 0.5 mile apart

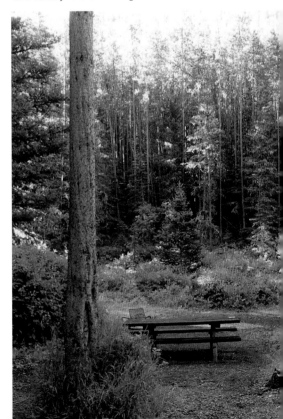

Swan Creek Campground provides peace and quiet in a densely forested setting.

ADDRESS: Swan Creek Road (Forest Road 421), Bozeman, MT 59718

CONTACT: 406-522-2520, www.fs.usda.gov /custergallatin; reservations: 877-444-6777, recreation.gov

OPERATED BY: Yellowstone Country Campgrounds

OPEN: Mid-May–September

SITES: 12

EACH SITE: Picnic table, fire grate

ASSIGNMENT: First come, first served and by reservation

REGISTRATION: On-site self-registration

FACILITIES: Hand-pump well, vault toilets

PARKING: At campsites

FEE: $15, $7/additional vehicle

ELEVATION: 5,800'

RESTRICTIONS:

Pets: On leash only

Fires: In fire rings only

Alcohol: Permitted

Vehicles: 55-foot length limit; 2 vehicles/site

Other: 16-day stay limit; bear-country food storage restrictions

along the creek. Sites in the first section are a bit farther from the creek than ones in the second, but all are well buffered with thick understory, and they have the best access to the hand pump. Sites 1 and 2 are the nonreservable sites in this section, and they are comparable to the other four in terms of size and privacy.

The sites in the second section are preferred because they all back up to the creek and have a narrow trail leading to the water. The understory here is thick as well, providing privacy and blocking your view of neighboring sites. Sites 7 and 8 are nonreservable. Our favorites are sites 10 and 12, which are particularly well suited for tenters, with the picnic table and fire ring up closer to the parking spur and spacious areas near the creek for your tent. No water is available here; you'll have to hike up to the first section.

A tidy, peaceful campsite situated next to a babbling brook

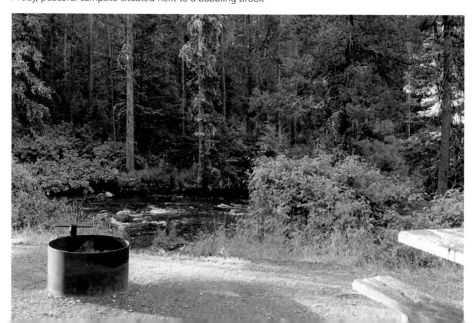

The creek itself is no more than 10–15 feet across, but it offers the same variety of fish as the Gallatin for those looking to hone their skills. If you're seeking other ways to relax, the thick streamside vegetation makes it easy to find a quiet place to set your chair while you lose yourself in a good book or take out a sketchpad and pencils.

Just down the road from the last site is the trailhead for Swan Creek Trail #186. This 2-mile trail is great for families or those who want a stroll instead of a strenuous hike. The route winds along the creek to the base of Hyalite Peak (10,298'). Dozens of trails, both to the east and west, are accessible off US 191. A major trailhead lies 6 miles south of the Swan Creek Road turnoff and then 6 miles east on Portal Creek Road (FR 984). From there, you can take an easy hike to Golden Trout Lakes or a steep, challenging hike to Windy Pass. Additional trails interconnect and provide options to please everyone.

Swan Creek Campground

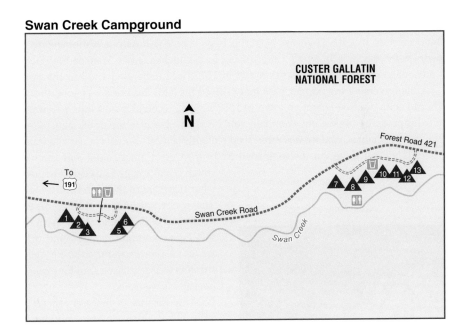

GETTING THERE

From Bozeman, take US 191 south for 32 miles to Swan Creek Road (FR 421). Turn left and go 1 mile east to the campground.

GPS COORDINATES: N45° 22.412' W111° 9.164'

37

Tom Miner Campground

Beauty: ★★★★ / Privacy: ★★★★ / Quiet: ★★★★ / Spaciousness: ★★★★ / Security: ★★★ /
Cleanliness: ★★★

A dense mix of firs and aspens provides plenty of shade in summer and vibrant color in autumn.

Winding alongside the Yellowstone River through the aptly named Paradise Valley, US 89 from Livingston to this campground's turnoff is one of the most scenic in the state. With the Absaroka Mountains to the east and the Gallatin peaks to the west, even views from the roadway are incredible. Fly-fishing and floating are the draw for this stretch of river, and scores of multimillion-dollar ranches attract the rich and famous.

Access to this area hasn't always been this easy. When Yellowstone National Park first opened, US 89 was merely a trail. Enterprising local rancher James "Yankee Jim" George took advantage of his strategic location and in 1872 began charging a toll to the miners and wagons traversing the narrow pass that crossed his land. Business was good until the Northern Pacific Railroad came to town in 1883 seeking to build a spur into Yellowstone. Despite his protests, Yankee Jim eventually sold his right-of-way to the developing railroad, but his anger remained, and he was often seen violently shaking his fists at passing trains.

There is no toll today on the long road to Tom Miner Campground, but the road's rough condition gives campers a sense of what travelers in the 19th century faced. The rocky washboard surface discourages most RVs from making the trek to this high-mountain campground, which serves as a jumping-off point for Yellowstone as well as a base camp for exploring nearby hiking trails.

A dense mix of firs and aspens provides plenty of shade from summer heat and vibrant color in the autumn, while the elevation makes for cool nights and the possibility of snow year-round. Sites are perfect for tents (but see note at end of Key Information, opposite) and provide sufficient seclusion from other campers. A hand pump provides fresh drinking water, and a small creek running through the campground enhances mountain views.

Even though U.S. Forest Service information indicates that there are 16 sites here, just 12 are currently designated. The best ones are the 4 on the left side of the

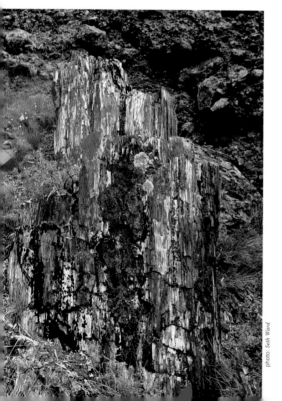

Petrified stump in Gallatin Petrified Forest

photo: *Seth Ward*

KEY INFORMATION

ADDRESS: Tom Miner Road (County Road 63), Gardiner, MT 59030

CONTACT: 406-848-7375, www.fs.usda.gov /custergallatin

OPERATED BY: Custer Gallatin National Forest, Gardiner Ranger District

OPEN: June–October, weather permitting

SITES: 12

EACH SITE: Picnic table, fire grate; bear-resistant boxes at most sites

ASSIGNMENT: First come, first served; no reservations

REGISTRATION: On-site self-registration

FACILITIES: Hand-pump well, vault toilets

PARKING: At campsites

FEE: $7, $3/additional vehicle

ELEVATION: 7,300'

RESTRICTIONS:

Pets: On leash only

Fires: In fire rings only

Alcohol: Permitted

Vehicles: 42-foot length limit

Other: 16-day stay limit; bear-country food storage restrictions; pack in, pack out. *Note:* At press time, the U.S. Forest Service was considering limiting the campground to hard-sided pop-up campers and RVs, so call or check online for the latest information.

road: 5, 7, 8, and 10. These sites are the largest and provide the most seclusion since they're backed by a dense stand of trees.

A unique hiking opportunity exists from the campground trailhead. An easy 2-mile hike takes you back thousands of years as you travel the Gallatin Petrified Forest Interpretive Trail #286. This trail loops from the campground and includes signs that describe the volcanic activity that occurred 44–53 million years ago, forever preserving this tropical forest. Many of the trees are preserved in an upright position, which raised a debate about whether they were petrified in place or transported and deposited in this position. Recent studies, which included looking at the aftermath of the 1980 eruption of Mount St. Helens, have led researchers to question their previous conclusions. See what conclusions you come to as you explore this prehistoric forest oasis.

Please keep in mind that collecting petrified wood along this trail is prohibited. You are, however, allowed to collect one small fragment elsewhere in the 25,000 acres designated as the Gallatin Petrified Forest. Just be sure to obtain a permit from the self-service permit station at the Gardiner Ranger District office, located at 805 Scott St. in Gardiner.

The trail to Buffalo Horn Pass also starts at this trailhead. This moderately easy 5-mile out-and-back hike follows Trail Creek as it gently climbs to the 8,523-foot summit. Along the way, many additional trails spur off into the Petrified Forest for further exploration.

If you continue on to Yellowstone National Park from here, be sure to stop at the Boiling River, about 2 miles south of the north entrance of the park. A short trail leads down to this spot in the Gardner River, where hot pools and small waterfalls provide a relaxing swimming area.

As you travel throughout Tom Miner Basin, you'll be in the company of both grizzly bears and one of the West's most controversial canines. Gray wolves inhabit this area after having been reintroduced to the Greater Yellowstone Ecosystem between 1995 and 1996. This reclusive predator was the center of a heated controversy between the ranching community and those interested in restoring this subspecies of the native Northern Rocky Mountain wolf. The wolves in this area have been busy reproducing, and area ranchers have lost livestock and pets to wolf kills. Efforts to prevent wolf–livestock encounters have been undertaken to compensate ranchers for their losses.

Additional wildlife-viewing opportunities are abundant, with white-tailed and mule deer, bighorn sheep, antelope, and elk frequently visiting the area; moose and grizzly bears visit too, but not nearly as often.

Tom Miner Campground

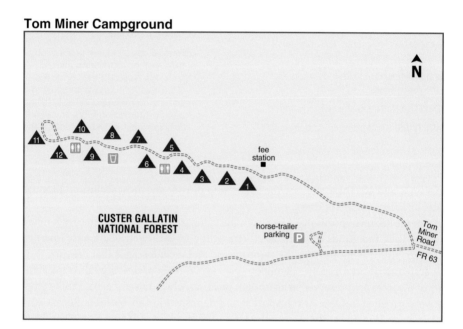

GETTING THERE

From Gardiner, take US 89 north for 16 miles to Tom Miner Road/Forest Road 63. Turn left and follow the campground signs 12 miles southwest to the campground.

GPS COORDINATES: N45° 7.763' W111° 3.752'

38

Wade and Cliff Lakes Area Campgrounds

Beauty: ★★★★★ / Privacy: ★★★★ / Quiet: ★★★★ / Spaciousness: ★★★★ / Security: ★★★★★ / Cleanliness: ★★★★★

The cliffs surrounding these mountain lakes are home to prairie falcons, bald eagles, and osprey.

The Madison Valley stretches about 60 miles north to south and is bordered by the Gravelly Range to the west and the Madison Range to the east. Right down the middle runs a ribbon of world-class trout-laden river. This scenery is outstanding largely because of the area's location along the western edge of the Madison fault line, with the most active section of the fault line lying beneath the waters of Wade and Cliff Lakes.

Today the lakes' waters are calm and serene, but in 1959, aftershocks from the Hebgen Lake earthquake measured between 5.8 and 6.0 on the Richter scale, and Wade Lake campers awoke thinking bears were shaking their trailers. That is, until they and their trailers began to bounce 3 feet off the ground and they watched the lake slosh like a giant bucket of water, tossing fish and debris up onto its banks.

On the drive in, you'd never guess these lakes were here. You leave the highway, cross the Madison River, and drive across seemingly endless views of sagebrush. You pass the ghost town of Cliff Lake and see cabin remnants, but nowhere is there anything resembling a lake. One more hill climb, and suddenly everything changes. The flats begin to roll and the transformation between sagebrush prairie and forest begins. Around the final bend are these two mountain lakes, shimmering in the distance.

Part of the Hidden Lakes chain, both Cliff and Wade Lakes are surrounded by cliffs that make shoreline fishing difficult but provide excellent habitat for the prairie falcons, bald eagles, and osprey that call this area home. Once you get offshore, fishing here is a delight. Experts and novices use a variety of styles, from fly-fishing to spin casting to trolling from canoes, drift boats, and float tubes, and the no-wake rules keep noise and activity at manageable levels.

A spawning channel has been installed to eliminate the need for annual stocking, and it's surprising more anglers don't visit here. The state-record brown trout (29 pounds) was caught at Wade Lake, and Cliff Lake was home to the state-record

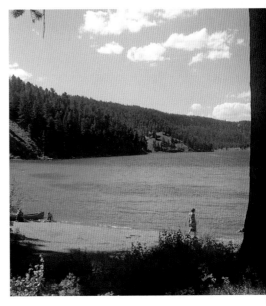

Wade and Cliff Lakes provide waterside camping and superb trout fishing.

KEY INFORMATION

ADDRESS: Wade Lake Road (Forest Road 8381), Ennis, MT 59729

CONTACT: 406-682-4253 or 406-682-7560, www.fs.usda.gov/bdnf

OPERATED BY: Beaverhead-Deerlodge National Forest, Madison Ranger District (Dave and Laurie Schmidt, concessionaires)

OPEN: Whenever accessible; water available June–Labor Day only

SITES: 54

EACH SITE: Picnic table, fire grate

ASSIGNMENT: First come, first served; no reservations. Note that you may need to arrive midweek to secure a site over the weekend during summer.

REGISTRATION: On-site self-registration

FACILITIES: Water spigots, vault toilets, boat launch

PARKING: At campsites

FEE: $15

ELEVATION: 6,217'

RESTRICTIONS:

Pets: On leash only

Fires: In fire rings only

Alcohol: Permitted

Vehicles: 24-foot length limit

Other: 16-day stay limit; bear-country food storage restrictions; no-wake boating restrictions

rainbow trout for over 35 years. Fish are plentiful, and when lake fishing becomes boring, you'll find several blue-ribbon trout streams within a short drive.

The water is a crystal-clear emerald with huge boulders visible beneath the surface, hiding healthy populations of crayfish. Cliff Lake is more isolated. Its long and narrow shape is a flatwater paddler's dream, with coves to investigate and plenty of places to pull ashore and explore. If you don't have a boat, don't worry. Rentals are available from Wade Lake Cabins at the south end of Wade Lake.

There are three separate campgrounds: Wade Lake, Cliff Point, and Hilltop. A favorite is at Wade Lake, with 30 sites from which to choose, great lake access, and two of the best public campsites in this area. It would be hard to find a better site than one of these walk-in sites without strapping on a backpack and hiking boots. You can access both walk-in sites from the northwest corner of the parking area near the boat launch. Marked with an inconspicuous sign, these treasured sites are about 50 yards from the parking lot. Both spacious

Walk-in tent sites at Wade Lake are accessed from the parking area near the boat launch.

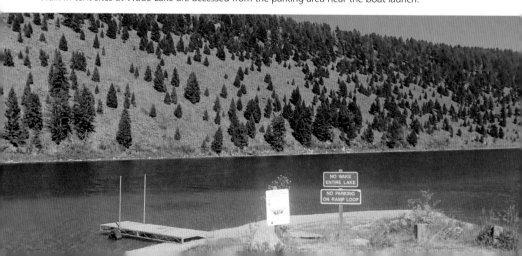

sites overlook the lake and are fairly well hidden from the rest of the campground. Another perk for those lucky enough to snag one of these sites is access to a trail leading to the rocky shoreline and a perfect place to park your canoe or just enjoy your surroundings.

If the tent-only sites are not available, there are many other great choices among the remaining 28. Head for the northwest corner of the loop and choose one of the sites on the outer edge of the loop for views of the lake. These sites should be quieter than the others, but they are a bit tight. With a little ingenuity you'll be set up and enjoying the serenity in no time.

The smallest campground of the trio is Cliff Point, with six campsites on Cliff Lake. All sites sit in the open with little shade, and views from each are grand. The road is rougher here, and the sites are loosely defined, but each does have a picnic table and fire ring. The campground has a single vault toilet and a water spigot.

Hilltop offers 18 nicely spaced campsites set in a mixture of pines and fir. Sites vary, with some offering great shade cover and others partially open to the sun, wind, and views. From Hilltop, a 0.7-mile interpretive trail winds to Wade Lake Campground. Information about the flora, fauna, and geology of the area is only the beginning, since you'll also see plenty of wildlife. Moose, in particular, are frequently observed along the lakeshores at dusk and in the early morning.

Wade and Cliff Lakes Area Campgrounds

GETTING THERE

From Ennis, take US 287 south for 39.5 miles to Forest Road 8381. Turn right and go 6 miles to Wade Lake Campground.

GPS COORDINATES: N45° 48.436′ W111° 33.971′

39

West Fork Madison Dispersed Sites

Beauty: ★★★★★ / Privacy: ★★★★ / Quiet: ★★★★ / Spaciousness: ★★★★★ / Security: ★★★★ /
Cleanliness: ★★★

This string of little-known campsites sits along an out-of-the-way road.

Tucked behind a natural rise and isolated from the neoprene-clad anglers on the Madison River is an out-of-the-way road lined with little-known campgrounds. Just off MT 287, you'll discover this scenic back road where secluded campgrounds are spread along the West Fork of the Madison River. The West Fork Madison River runs cool, clear, and fast from the Gravelly Range to where it dumps into the Madison River at Lyons Bridge. Brown and rainbow trout are plentiful, but they're smart—they've had lots of practice outfoxing wily anglers.

Fishing the West Fork or the Madison itself is far different than it was in the late 1980s. Back then counts of more than 3,000 rainbow trout per mile were not uncommon, and some days drift boats far outnumbered the cars along the highway. But when whirling disease (a sickness in fish caused by a parasite called *Myxobolus cerebralis*) came to Montana, it hit the Madison and its branches first. The rainbow population was the hardest hit, dwindling to less than 20 percent of its previous number. With strong mitigation efforts, a flood of educational material for anglers and boaters, and impressive research results, the rainbows have made an impressive comeback, with reports indicating the population approaching 2,000 rainbows per mile.

The five dispersed campsites provide plenty of space and privacy, beautiful views, and access to fishing but no water, metal fire rings, or picnic tables, and not all have vault toilets. Each site is marked with a 4-foot-tall, 4-inch-wide fiberglass post with a tent-camping symbol and number near the top. These designate the turnoffs for the individual sites. If you're heading to one of these sites, be familiar with low-impact camping practices to

These dispersed sites provide plenty of seclusion, elbow room, and natural beauty.

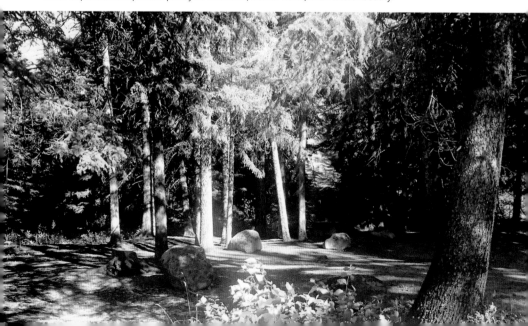

KEY INFORMATION

ADDRESS: West Fork Madison Road
(Forest Road 209), Ennis, MT 59729

CONTACT: 406-682-4253 or 406-682-7560,
www.fs.usda.gov/bdnf

OPERATED BY: Beaverhead-Deerlodge
National Forest, Madison Ranger District
(Dave and Laurie Schmidt, concessionaires)

OPEN: June–mid-September

SITES: 5

EACH SITE: Rock fire ring

ASSIGNMENT: First come, first served;
no reservations

REGISTRATION: None

FACILITIES: Vault toilets at some sites;
no other facilities

PARKING: At campsites

FEE: Free

ELEVATION: 6,000'

RESTRICTIONS:

Pets: On leash only

Fires: In fire rings only

Alcohol: Permitted

Vehicles: RVs not advised

Other: 16-day stay limit; bear-country
food storage restrictions; pack in,
pack out; no cell phone coverage

reduce your footprint on the land. Also note that access to most of these sites can get rutted in wet weather.

Site 1, which lies on the east side of the road, is bordered by cottonwoods and lies very near the water, with beautiful views of several 9,000-foot peaks to the west and the Madison Range to the east. Site 2 sits along the West Fork in a serene and peaceful spot with plenty of space to spread out. Site 3 is a beautiful site in a delightful setting in a shady grove secluded from the road. Site 4 is another gem with great river access, plenty of shade, and enough flat ground to make finding a place to rest your head under a star-soaked Montana sky a cinch. Site 5 sits on the west side of the road in a large open area, but you'll find shade along the edge of the tree line.

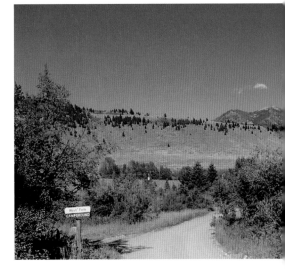

Should all the dispersed sites be taken, turn your vehicle around and try the West Fork Madison Campground near Lyons Bridge.

If the dispersed sites are full, head back toward the highway and try one of the seven sites at West Fork Madison Campground ($12 fee). You'll still have great access to the river, but you'll sacrifice the privacy offered by a dispersed site.

With the Gravelly Range basically out your back door to the west, if you're up for a scenic drive the Gravelly Range Road Backcountry Drive is 72 miles of bliss. It's been called the most scenic drive in Montana, with sweeping views of the entire Beaverhead-Deerlodge National Forest and Madison Valley area. The route crosses an expansive high-elevation plateau through the heart of the Gravelly Range, where a visit from late June through July can offer electric sights of fields of brilliant wildflower blooms. You'll need a map to know how to connect the route to or from Ennis, although access can be gained from the campground by driving south on Forest Road 209.

West Fork Madison Dispersed Sites

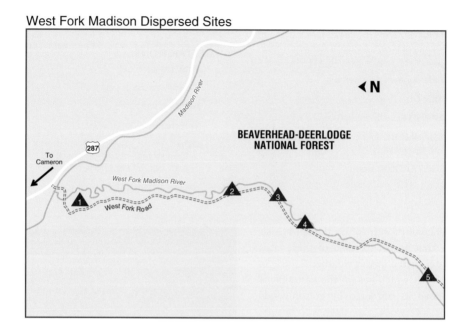

GETTING THERE

From Ennis, take US 287 south for 34 miles. Turn right on West Fork Road and head west. Cross the river and watch for campsite markers.

GPS COORDINATES: N44° 53.213' W111° 34.931'

SOUTHWEST MONTANA

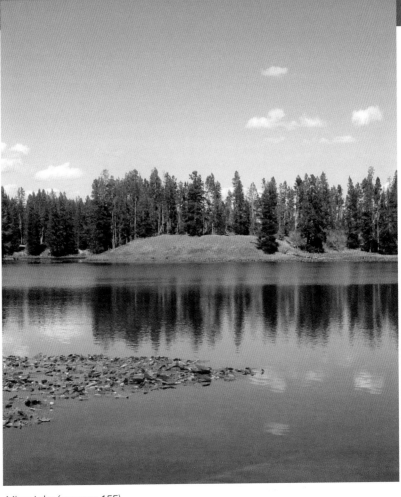

Miner Lake *(see page 155)*

40

Bannack State Park Campground

Beauty: ★★★★ / Privacy: ★★★★ / Quiet: ★★★★★ / Spaciousness: ★★★★ / Security: ★★★★★ /
Cleanliness: ★★★★★

Claim your site in this ghost town once called "the toughest town in the West."

A nondescript guideboard with letters scratched into it was nailed to a post along a rutted road. It reads, TU GRASSHOPPER DIGNS 30 MYLE KEEP THE TRALE NEX THE BLUFFE. This simple message led hundreds of hopeful gold prospectors to Grasshopper Creek, where they expected to find gold just as John White did in July of 1862. Within 10 months, the population swelled to over 5,000, but, like a typical boomtown, it had only a few hundred people left by 1865.

The town was named Bannack, a misspelling of the name for the local Bannock tribe. This was Montana's first territorial capital, its gold bringing more than miners, as others saw potential to make their "pile" offering goods and services to those seeking their fortunes with a pick and a pan.

Men like Sidney Edgerton, Granville Stuart, and Wilbur Fisk Sanders arrived here and left their mark on Montana history in ways far beyond the riches of gold. Others, like Henry Plummer, left their mark due to greed and lawlessness. Their stories and those of countless others are recounted here by the interpretive staff, informational and interactive programs, self-guided tours, signs, and brochures.

If you love history, then you'll love Bannack. This town has it all—gold mining, politics, lawlessness, romance, vigilantes, boom, and bust—and presents it in an atmospheric package that retains its dusty streets and weathered buildings. Rather than being developed and commercialized, it exists in a state of arrested decay, allowing visitors to explore the abandoned

Bannack was Montana's first territorial capital.

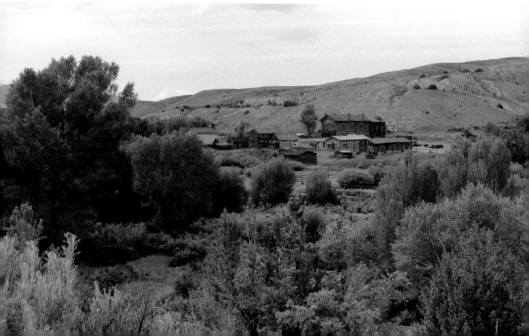

KEY INFORMATION

ADDRESS: 721 Bannack Road, Dillon, MT 59725

CONTACT: 406-834-3413, stateparks.mt.gov /bannack; reservations: reserveamerica.com

OPERATED BY: Bannack State Park

OPEN: Year-round when accessible; full services Memorial Day weekend–Labor Day

SITES: 24

EACH SITE: Picnic table, fire grate

ASSIGNMENT: First come, first served or by reservation

REGISTRATION: On-site self-registration or at visitor center (when open)

FACILITIES: Water, vault toilets, tepee, visitor center, firewood for sale

PARKING: At campsites

FEE: $18 resident, $28 nonresident; $6/extra nonresident vehicle

ELEVATION: 5,837′

RESTRICTIONS:

Pets: On leash only

Fires: In fire rings only

Alcohol: Permitted

Vehicles: 60-foot length limit

Other: 14-day stay limit

---

buildings in ghostly silence and create for themselves a picture of what life in the "toughest town in the West" must have been like.

Most of the buildings are open to the public. Some of the most well preserved include the Meade Hotel (formerly the Beaverhead County Courthouse), the Methodist Church, the Masonic Lodge with its first-floor schoolhouse, and the home of Fielding L. Graves (developer of the first electric gold dredge). Investigating the nooks and crannies can take hours, and a short hike along the gravel road up past the mill to Yankee Flats provides an unspoiled view of Main Street, which has barely changed in over a century. For a more structured experience, stop at the visitor center and see the video on

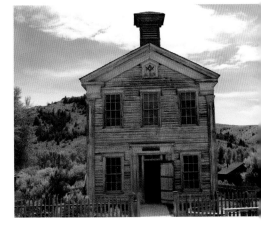

Bannack's Masonic Lodge

Henry Plummer's stash of gold, which has never been found. Interpretive programs are provided throughout the summer, and the third weekend in July brings the park alive with a full-scale living-history event.

The campground at Bannack sits along a creek originally named Willard by the Lewis and Clark Expedition in 1805. In 1862, the creek was nicknamed Grasshopper due to the healthy population of the insect along its banks, and the name stuck. The creek's clear water contains cagey brown trout that may prove elusive unless tempted with the smooth cast of a carefully matched fly.

Tent sites along the creek are the choicest in the campground. There are actually two separate areas: Vigilante and Road Agent. The former is named after an impromptu group of folks who took the law into their own hands to control the latter, a lawless group who scammed, robbed, and murdered unsuspecting miners for their gold dust.

We prefer Vigilante, which hugs the creek and offers sites well separated from one another. Mature cottonwoods provide shade from the same high-noon heat that must have made creekside prospecting a welcome occupation compared with the subsequent hard-rock mining efforts on the surrounding hillsides, especially when the easy pickings from the creek played out. These sites provide a great place for a night of stargazing, with the ghosts of Bannack adding an interesting twist to your evening campfire stories.

As is the case with so many other places in Montana, the weather here can be extreme. The elevation is deceiving, since there aren't lofty mountain peaks (or many trees) nearby, but be prepared for scorching heat or subfreezing temperatures no matter what the weather report says.

If you're looking for something a little different, consider leaving your tent in the trunk and trying the tepee that's available for rent at the campground. Large enough to fit six comfortably, it will take you on a journey to the days before gold was discovered and the riches of the area were found in the distant call of a coyote or ghostly hoot of an owl.

Bannack State Park Campground

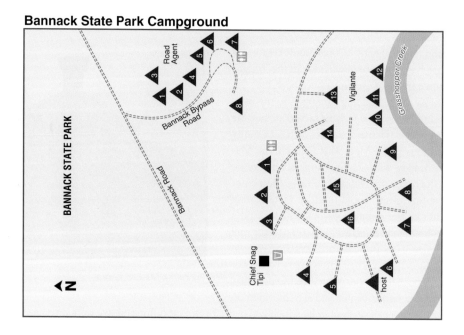

GETTING THERE

From Dillon, take I-15 south to Exit 59 and go 17 miles west on MT 278. Turn left at the park sign and go 4 miles south to the campground.

GPS COORDINATES: N45° 9.895′ W113° 0.252′

41

Charles Waters Campground

Beauty: ★★★★ / Privacy: ★★★★ / Quiet: ★★★★ / Spaciousness: ★★★★ / Security: ★★★★★ /
Cleanliness: ★★★★★

Even if you don't snag a creekside site, you'll still be able to enjoy the sound of water cascading over trees and rocks.

This campground sits within the Bass Creek Recreation Area, a multiuse area designed for hikers, equestrians, and mountain bikers to peacefully coexist—and most of the time it works pretty well. If you are not lucky enough to snag one of the creekside sites, you can still enjoy the sound of water cascading over trees and rocks.

Sites 12, 18, 20, 22, and 25 are the best, providing you with a creekside stay and a spur trail leading to the water. Bass Creek is narrow here, and the water is clear, enabling you to see the cutthroat trout even though there are a lot of trees lying in the creekbed to provide cover for them. It may be wise to steer clear of sites 13 and 15, at the end of the loop road, unless you have a large group or don't mind being close to one. The sign in front of site 14 indicates its capacity is between 12 and 20, and a large open field in front is perfect for throwing Frisbees or playing a noisy game of softball.

A second campground, Larry Creek, is 1 mile down the road and part of the Bass Creek Recreation Area. This group-only area, set in a stand of mature trees, may be one of the nicest U.S. Forest Service group sites in the state. If you're still looking for a site, this might be your answer. On the road into Larry Creek, on your right before you get to the campground, a couple of secret sites are tucked on a short spur road. It's easy to miss them, but they're well maintained and provide fire rings and tables. As long as you don't mind a short trek to Charles Waters to get water and use the restrooms, you'll be in great shape.

An extensive network of trails lies within the recreation area, with many of these trails leading into the adjacent Selway-Bitterroot Wilderness. A short spur leads from the campground to Bass Creek Scenic Overlook and is a great way to start the day. From here, Trail #392 is a 3-mile ridge trail. Those seeking education can choose the 0.5-mile nature trail. Another interpretive trail, the 2.5-mile fire-ecology loop, provides information about the initial impact and long-term effects of fires in the forest.

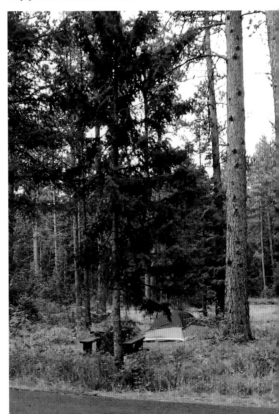

Tall, mature timber shelters a tenter at Charles Waters, where hikers, equestrians and mountain bikers can enjoy an abundance of trails.

KEY INFORMATION

ADDRESS: Bass Creek Road, Stevensville, MT 59870

CONTACT: 406-777-5461, www.fs.usda.gov /bitterroot

OPERATED BY: Bitterroot National Forest, Stevensville Ranger District

OPEN: May–September

SITES: 25

EACH SITE: Picnic table, fire grate

ASSIGNMENT: First come, first served; no reservations

REGISTRATION: On-site self-registration

FACILITIES: Water spigots, vault toilets

PARKING: At campsites

FEE: $10

ELEVATION: 3,690'

RESTRICTIONS:

Pets: On leash only

Fires: In fire rings only

Alcohol: Permitted

Vehicles: 70-foot length limit

Other: 16-day stay limit; bear-country food-storage precautions recommended

The fire-ecology trail extends into the 6.5-mile day-use trail that offers a gentle hike and several spurs, so you create an individualized route. Hawks, deer, and great horned owls are frequently seen here, as are mountain bluebirds.

The day-use and fire-ecology trails are open to horses and mountain bikes as well as hikers, so if you're looking for a more serious hike, try Bass Creek Trail #4, a 16.8-mile round-trip along the creek to Bass Lake. Mountain bikes may share the trail for the first 2.5 miles, but at that point the trail enters the Selway-Bitterroot Wilderness, where bicycles are prohibited. From this point you will still see horses, but probably not as many. Along this segment, the canyon begins to gradually narrow as you are treated to meadow views, rare in the Bitterroot forest, and several gentle waterfalls. The lake itself nestles in a deep canyon, and anglers can try their luck at catching rainbow and cutthroat trout.

Four miles south on US 93 is Kootenai Creek Road. Drive 2 miles west to find the trailhead for Kootenai Creek Trail #53. This well-used trail parallels the route of Trail 4 but follows Kootenai Creek to North and South Kootenai Lakes. Another option is the 4.5-mile hike to St. Mary Peak Lookout #116, which begins south of Stevensville off St. Mary's Peak Road.

To the east of Stevensville is Lee Metcalf National Wildlife Refuge. Named for a long-time Montana senator who grew up in the area, the refuge provides nearly 3 miles of nature trails that wind through river bottoms and meadows. A short paved path leads through the wildlife-viewing area to a scenic spot on the Bitterroot River, and there is also a scenic drive along Wildfowl Lane that runs the length of the refuge. Bald eagles and osprey nest here, and more than 100 other species are on the confirmed nester list.

In the middle of it all is the state's oldest town, Stevensville (population 1,809). It was here in 1841 that Father Pierre DeSmet established St. Mary's Mission. The mission's early years were fruitful, but by 1850 the missionaries decided to close the mission temporarily. At the same time, Philadelphia native John Owen arrived in the area and took over the mission site, building a trading post and fort. It would be 16 years before the missionaries returned to build a new mission. The "new" mission complex still stands and is open for tours during spring and summer, while the remains of John Owen's trading post are now owned by the state and preserved as Fort Owen State Park.

Charles Waters Campground

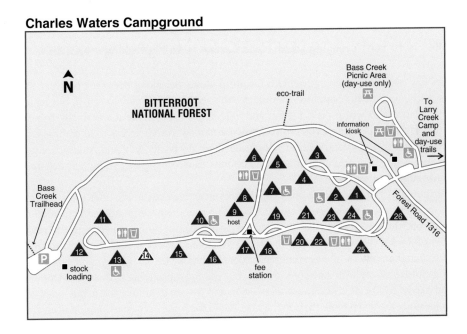

GETTING THERE

From Missoula, take US 93 south for 25 miles. Turn left (west) on Bass Creek Road (County Road 20) and go 2 miles to the campground. Look for the parking area on Forest Road 1316.

From Stevensville, take US 93 north for 5 miles. Turn right (west) on Bass Creek Road (CR 20) and go 2 miles to the campground. Look for the parking area on FR 1316.

GPS COORDINATES: N46° 34.516' W114° 8.450'

42

⛺ Dalles Campground

Beauty: ★★★★ / Privacy: ★★★★ / Quiet: ★★★★★ / Spaciousness: ★★★★ / Security: ★★★ / Cleanliness: ★★★★

Dalles is to tent camping what Rock Creek is to fly fishing—paradise.

Dalles is a tent-camping paradise with beautiful views. Set along the creek between steep cliffs, with views of the Sapphire Mountains, this campground may be small, but its location and access to world-class fishing and wilderness areas make it worth the trip. And the trip to Dalles isn't easy; you'll travel down a narrow, rough access road complete with hairpin turns and one-lane sections alongside sheer drop-offs. July and August are prime time here, since the somewhat marshy conditions caused by spring snowmelt dry up and the mosquitoes move on.

With only 10 sites, Dalles is often full, but if you arrive early in the afternoon, especially on a weekday, you'll have a good chance of getting a site. The setting is perfect: steep cliffs rising from the forest floor, views of rugged peaks waiting to be scaled, and the rushing waters of Rock Creek calling below. Each site overlooks the creek, and while some are better situated than others, all have unique features that make them a grand choice for tenting.

Campsites sit on both sides of the road, but the most desirable sites are the three with direct access to Rock Creek. These sites—4, 6, and 8—are definitely the prime ones, since they lie along the steep bank that can be negotiated for some early-morning or after-dinner casting. Parking for site 1 is right along the road. Pull off as far as you can and walk the hillside into this secluded little site, which offers a table, a fire ring, and an area to set up a small tent. Restrooms are right behind it. Sites on the opposite side of the road from the creek have the advantage of sitting on a slight rise above the road, giving them an added bit of privacy. And it still isn't too far or difficult to access the creek.

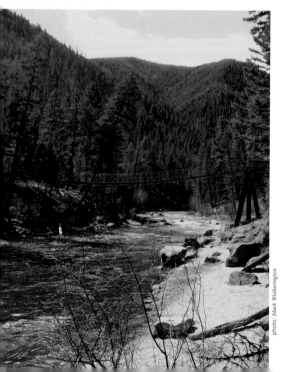

Swinging bridge in Welcome Creek Wilderness

photo: Mark Wetherington

Camping along Rock Creek and Forest Road 102 is limited to established campgrounds and a series of designated dispersed sites. Dalles is our pick as the best of the established spots, although several dispersed sites are found along Rock Creek. You are encouraged to try one, especially if there are no sites available here.

The fish in Rock Creek are cagey. Having been fished frequently, they've become quite mischievous, so a catch here takes skill, patience, and plenty of plain old luck. But who could ask for a

KEY INFORMATION

ADDRESS: Rock Creek Road
(Forest Road 102), Clinton, MT 59825

CONTACT: 406-329-3814,
www.fs.usda.gov/lolo

OPERATED BY: Lolo National Forest,
Missoula Ranger District

OPEN: Generally spring–fall, with fees
charged April–September

SITES: 10

EACH SITE: Picnic table, fire grate

ASSIGNMENT: First come, first served;
no reservations

REGISTRATION: On-site self-registration

FACILITIES: Water (variable), vault toilets

PARKING: At campsites; 2 vehicles/site

FEE: $6

ELEVATION: 4,200'

RESTRICTIONS:

Pets: On leash only

Fires: In fire rings only

Alcohol: Permitted

Vehicles: 30-foot length limit; RVs not
recommended due to access road

Other: 16-day stay limit; bear-country
food storage restrictions; pack in,
pack out

better competition arena? Abundant streamside undergrowth fills with wildflowers through-out the summer, and the scenery is spectacular.

Throughout the Rock Creek Corridor and elsewhere west of the Continental Divide, you may see small plastic items stapled 10–12 feet high on the tree trunks. Designed to be as unobtrusive as possible, they house repellents, as part of the U.S. Forest Service's response to bark-beetle infestations that have impacted hundreds of thousands of acres across the state. Ordinarily, the beetles feed on dead trees, but with the number of recent forest fires, much of the deadfall and undergrowth has been burnt out, so they've turned to live trees for food, taking a devastating toll on remaining forests. Trees under severe stress due to years of drought are unable to produce sap and natural repellents, so they easily fall prey.

A quarter mile north of Dalles is the Welcome Creek Wilderness trailhead. Trail #225 starts by crossing a suspension bridge over the creek and then follows the creek before climbing to the top of Cleveland Mountain. Additional trails cross the dramatic canyons, heavily forested slopes, and rocky ridges of this 29,000-acre designated wilderness area, but this is the most popular trailhead.

Gold was discovered in Welcome Creek in 1888, and placer mines quickly evolved and almost as quickly played out, but not before one of the largest gold nuggets ever found in the state—close to 1.5 pounds—was discovered. Following the miners were fugitives who took refuge in the steep terrain, establishing hideouts and disappearing into the wilderness. It has been over a century since the miners left, but the weathered remains of several cabins can still be found in unexpected spots across the landscape.

Two miles south of I-90 is the trailhead for the former Valley of the Moon Nature Trail, a half-mile level path that winds through a creekside grove of cottonwood trees and provides habitat for elk, deer, and a wealth of birds like red-naped sapsuckers and yellow warblers. While the trail is no longer maintained and parts of it and its bridges have washed away due to flooding and shifting of the main Rock Creek channel, amateur geologists will enjoy exploring this visual wonderland of sedimentary and volcanic rocks.

A few miles farther north is Babcock Mountain, an excellent spot for viewing the bighorn sheep that come here during their April–mid-June lambing seasons. An interpretive sign at the trailhead of Spring Creek Trail #91 describes what makes good bighorn sheep habitat, although the trail itself is closed from April 15 through June 7 during the spring lambing season.

Dalles Campground

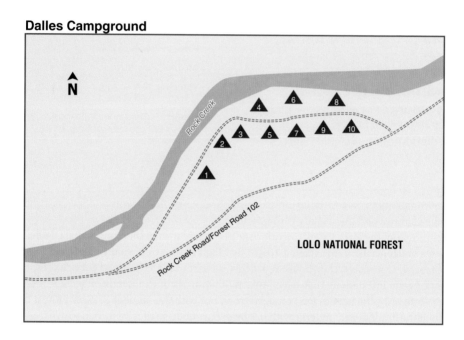

GETTING THERE

From Clinton, take I-90 east for 5 miles to Exit 126 for Rock Creek. Go south on FR 102 for 14.5 miles to the campground.

GPS COORDINATES: N46° 33.443' W113° 42.625'

43

△ Grasshopper Campground

Beauty: ★★★★★ / Privacy: ★★★★ / Quiet: ★★★★ / Spaciousness: ★★★★ / Security: ★★★★ / Cleanliness: ★★★★

Spacious creekside sites tucked at the bottom of steep canyon walls beckon campers.

Escape the paved roads you'll find at other campgrounds along the Pioneer Mountains National Scenic Byway by staying at this campground on the south end near Elkhorn Hot Springs. Snugly situated at the bottom of steep canyon walls, Grasshopper offers spacious sites, many of which lie right along the creek.

Pioneer Mountains National Scenic Byway, designated in 1989, is a picturesque ribbon of road winding between the 10,000-foot-plus peaks of the East Pioneers and the lower forested slopes of the West Pioneers. Fifty peaks exceed 10,000 feet, topping out with Mount Tweedy, at 11,154 feet in the eastern range. As close as these ranges are to one another, they bear little resemblance, with one gently rounded and the other sharply peaked. The difference lies in the amount of sandstone that has been eroded away from the granite surface below. Overall, the Pioneers are a rugged range dotted with lakes, laced with hiking trails, and well worth exploring.

Both Wise River and Grasshopper Creek weave from side to side along the highway, split by a 7,800-foot divide about halfway down the highway. The Wise River runs north, draining into Big Hole River near its namesake town, while Grasshopper Creek originates high in the mountains and runs south for 50 miles, passing through nearby Bannack State Park before emptying into the Beaverhead River. Fishing here focuses on brook, rainbow, and cutthroat trout.

The setting is peaceful, with the gentle sound of Grasshopper Creek, the lack of road noise, and the scent of pines providing idyllic surroundings. Sites 9–17 hug the creek bank and provide a great place to rest after a day of exploring all the area has to offer. Sites 9, 10, 11, and 12 are situated along the creek and offer a feeling of seclusion. If these sites are already taken, try sites 15, 16, or 17, and you will still be along the creek. Even if the creekside sites aren't available, any of the sites here will work; they're all spacious and suitable for tents.

A moderate walk from the campground to the northeast (you could take the car, but . . .) leads you to Elkhorn Hot Springs. The pools, built in 1918, offer hot waters to sooth tired, aching hiking muscles; while the facilities are rustic and basic, it's a charming step back to the 1920s, when wealthy tourists first discovered the region.

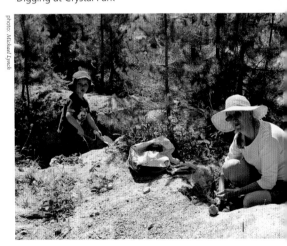

Digging at Crystal Park

photo: Michael Lynch

KEY INFORMATION

ADDRESS: Pioneer Mountains National Scenic Byway, Dillon, MT 59725

CONTACT: 406-683-3900, www.fs.usda.gov/bdnf

OPERATED BY: Beaverhead-Deerlodge National Forest, Dillon Ranger District

OPEN: Year-round when accessible; water available mid-June–mid-September only

SITES: 23

EACH SITE: Picnic table, fire ring

ASSIGNMENT: First come, first served; no reservations

REGISTRATION: On-site self-registration

FACILITIES: Water spigots, vault toilets

PARKING: At campsites

FEE: $8, $2/additional vehicle; free mid-September–mid-June

ELEVATION: 6,900'

RESTRICTIONS:

Pets: On leash only

Fires: In fire rings only

Alcohol: Permitted

Vehicles: 30-foot length limit

Other: 16-day stay limit; bear-country food storage restrictions; pack in, pack out

---

If you want to do some hiking, there is a trailhead 2 miles east of Elkhorn Hot Springs on Willman Creek Road (Forest Road 7441). Sawtooth Lake Trail #195 is an 8-mile out-and-back hike to a mountain lake where the unusual golden trout is the main draw. Some sections of this trail are a bit steep, but the switchbacks help.

The trailhead for Blue Creek Trail #425 is just north of Grasshopper. This 7-mile hike is fairly level and interesting enough to keep kids entertained (especially with all of the lovely creek crossings). For those seeking something more strenuous, Brown's Lake Trail #2 begins at Mono Creek Campground (just north of the hot springs). The trail will take you 6 miles up to Tahepia Lake—the key word here being *up*, with two sections containing most of the 2,500-foot elevation gain.

Riding the backbone of the West Pioneers is Pioneer Loop National Recreation Trail #750. This 35-mile loop can be accessed from various spur trails and is well worth the time and preparation needed for a few days of backpacking.

Eleven miles north of the campground is Crystal Park, one of the most unusual public-access sites operated by the U.S. Forest Service. Visitors are actually encouraged to dig for treasures beneath the soil, and daily throughout the summer you'll see visitors of all ages on their hands and knees, armed with hand trowels, searching for a cache of six-sided quartz crystals and amethyst.

An alternative to Grasshopper is a secluded site at Boulder Creek, located in about the center of the Byway. Drive to the end of the main campground road at the end of the loop. Look for the primitive road sign and bump your way about 1,500 feet along deep ruts. Just before the road turns to the right and starts to head uphill, you will find the site nestled among a stand of pines to your left, on the creek bank. This is a primitive site with no picnic table. Please use Leave No Trace practices, and take the time to walk to the main campground to use the restroom facilities.

Grasshopper Campground

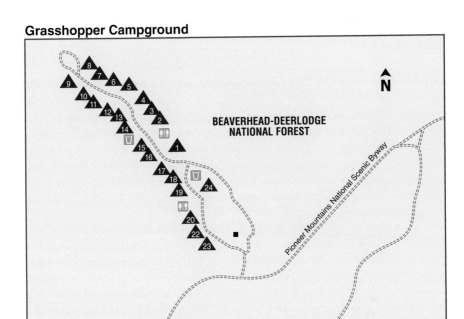

BEAVERHEAD-DEERLODGE NATIONAL FOREST

GETTING THERE

From MT 43 in Wise River, go south for 37.5 miles on the Pioneer Mountains National Scenic Byway to the campground.

From Dillon, take I-15 south for 3 miles to Exit 59, and go 27 miles west on MT 278 to the Pioneer Mountains National Scenic Byway. Turn right and go 11.5 miles north through Polaris to the campground.

GPS COORDINATES: N45° 27.045' W113° 7.121'

44

Lost Creek State Park Campground

Beauty: ★★★★ / Privacy: ★★★★ / Quiet: ★★★★ / Spaciousness: ★★★ / Security: ★★★★ / Cleanliness: ★★★★★

A crystal-clear creek in this narrow canyon creates an unexpected oasis.

A crystalline creek flows through this narrow canyon, creating an unexpected oasis in a landscape scarred by the mining fury of the past. Dwarfing the creekbed on either side are 1,200-foot limestone and granite walls, which provide habitat for mountain goats and bighorn sheep. Interpretive signs are strategically placed to educate visitors about the area's unique geology, which dates back 1.3 billion years. Colorful bands of gray and pink granite, originated as molten magma, forced its way into fissures and deposited a wealth of mineral resources.

This quiet place adjacent to the Beaverhead-Deerlodge National Forest and the town of Anaconda includes a 25-site campground that is split between sites on the upper and lower portions of the park road. The upper sites sit on an "island" at the end loop of the entrance road. The sites here are very tight, and only a few have a level spot on which to comfortably pitch a tent. Set on the inside of this loop, site 1 is roomy, with the tent and picnic area set slightly below the parking area. Site 6 is protected by large boulders and has plenty of level tent space but does sit very close to the road. Lost Creek Falls is visible from these sites, and a paved walking trail leads to the base of limestone cliffs below the 50-foot waterfall.

Sites 10, 11, and 12 run along the creek. Each is well shaded, has enough space to pitch a tent, and provides dramatic views of the towering rock walls. Mule deer and black bears frequent the area, particularly in spring, but it is the possibility of seeing bighorn sheep or mountain goats on the ledges or moose along the creek at dawn and dusk that's the main draw.

Mountain goats may also be visible from the designated pullout area where you enter the park. You might be fortunate enough to witness a pair of bighorn rams going at it like linebackers, but you'll probably hear the crashing of their horns long before you see them slamming into each other at full speed. Rocky Mountain bighorn sheep are well suited for the Lost Creek area. Their specially shaped hooves cling to the rock faces in ways that many rock climbers can only dream of, and their superior eyesight insures that they'll see you well before you focus your binoculars. The best viewing times are during winter and spring, although occasional summer sightings do occur.

The lower sites are well designed for tents, with extremely level and spacious

Sheer limestone cliffs

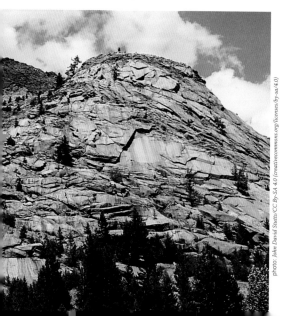

KEY INFORMATION

ADDRESS: 5750 Lost Creek Road, Anaconda, MT 59711

CONTACT: 406-287-3541, stateparks.mt.gov /lost-creek

OPERATED BY: Lost Creek State Park

OPEN: May–November

SITES: 25

EACH SITE: Picnic table, fire grate

ASSIGNMENT: First come, first served; no reservations

REGISTRATION: On-site self-registration

FACILITIES: Hand-pump well, vault toilets

PARKING: At campsites

FEE: $18 resident, $28 nonresident; $6/extra nonresident vehicle

ELEVATION: 6,000'

RESTRICTIONS:

Pets: On leash only

Fires: In fire rings only

Alcohol: Permitted

Vehicles: 23-foot length limit

Other: 14-day stay limit; bear-country food storage restrictions; pack in, pack out

layouts. These sites lack the views available from the upper campground, but they compensate with a creekside location. There are no designated parking pads here, so you may find vehicles parked somewhat haphazardly.

All campsites are located near the narrow park road; however, the thick understory and winding road help alleviate both noise and speeders. The temperature here is often cooler than in nearby Anaconda, since the window of direct sun during the day is severely limited by the shadows cast by the canyon walls.

Hiking is limited to an abandoned roadway near the end of the park road. This path meanders along the creek for 6 miles, making it a good out-and-back hike.

Mining is what brought this area to the world's attention back in the late 1800s. Anaconda, like Butte, began as a company town for copper magnate Marcus Daly, where he built the "Old Works" smelter to process ore from the Butte mines. Daly spent vast amounts of his own money enticing Montana voters to establish Anaconda as the state capital in 1894, but it wasn't enough. The city of Helena, backed by Daly's rival copper baron William Clark, won the title by 2,000 votes.

All that remains of the "Lower Works," built in 1889, is the smelter stack. At 585 feet, it is one of the world's tallest free-standing brick structures and is protected as a state park. With the mines came pollution of both the land and the water. A century later, Anaconda is one of many communities continuing to deal with the aftermath, but they've put an unusual twist on the reclamation process. Corporate, state, and federal cooperation enabled this site to become the Old Works Golf Course, a Jack Nicklaus signature course, where many of the remaining structures have been incorporated as an integral part of the world-class design.

A 1.5-mile, paved interpretive trail in Anaconda climbs above the town to provide an eagle's-eye view of the landscape's mining legacy. Also to the south is Fairmont Hot Springs, a year-round resort with Olympic-size hot pools and soaking pools both indoors and out, along with an outdoor water slide. Day passes are available, and it makes a great alternative for rainy, cold days.

Lost Creek State Park Campground

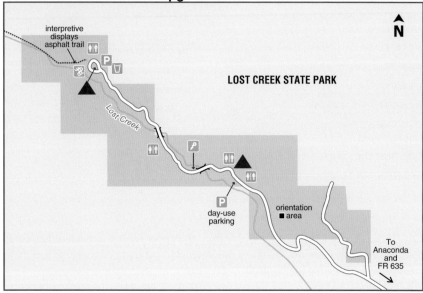

GETTING THERE

From Exit 208 off I-90, go 5.6 miles west toward Anaconda on MT 1 to MT 48. Turn right and go 0.25 mile to MT 273. Turn left and go north 2 miles to Forest Road 635. Turn left and go northwest for 7 miles to the campground. (The last 3 miles of FR 635 are gravel.)

From Anaconda, drive 2 miles east on MT 1 to MT 48. Turn right and go 0.25 mile to MT 273. Turn left and go north 2 miles to Forest Road 635. Turn left and go northwest for 7 miles to the campground. (The last 3 miles of FR 635 are gravel.)

GPS COORDINATES: N46° 12.559' W113° 0.202'

45

Martin Creek Campground

Beauty: ★★★★ / Privacy: ★★★ / Quiet: ★★★ / Spaciousness: ★★★★ / Security: ★★★ /
Cleanliness: ★★★★★

As you drive toward the campground, watch for the bighorn sheep herd at Angle Draw.

If you head toward Martin Creek in the early evening, stay alert and you may be in for a special treat. About 5 miles east of Sula is Angle Draw, the year-round home to a large herd of bighorn sheep. Viewing these hills above the East Fork Bitterroot River is a delight as the setting sun hits the hillside just so, and the glowing light makes the sheep even more visible.

You'll find the Broad Axe Lodge nearby. Initially, you might not be too impressed by the prospect of a restaurant in the middle of nowhere, but don't make the mistake of passing it up. The Broad Axe serves hearty Western fare, and every table comes with a pair of binoculars. These come in handy, since the expansive window-wall overlooks Angle Draw, and diners can watch sheep, deer, and elk and maybe glimpse an occasional bear.

The landscape around you may seem familiar. This valley is the setting for Charlie Russell's impressive 25-by-12-foot painting *Lewis and Clark Meeting Indians at Ross' Hole,* which hangs in the Montana State Capitol.

You could roll into Martin Creek late on a Saturday in mid-August and still have your pick of several sites. That's the beauty of Montana's southwestern corner: there are many campgrounds and dispersed sites from which to choose. Bordered by both Martin and Moose Creeks, the campground offers plenty of water frontage for everyone. Site 5 is a favorite, located on the back of the loop for privacy, and the sound of Moose Creek 10 yards away is quite inviting.

McCart Lookout

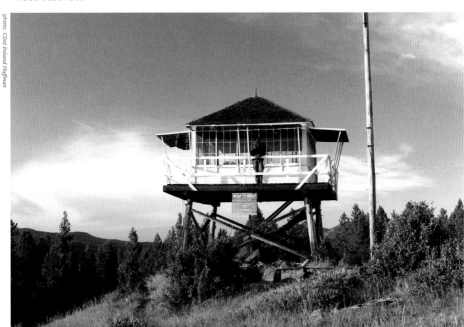

photo: *Clint Ireland Hoffman*

KEY INFORMATION

ADDRESS: Forest Road 726, Sula, MT 59871

CONTACT: 406-821-3913, www.fs.usda.gov
/bitterroot

OPERATED BY: Bitterroot National Forest,
Sula Ranger District

OPEN: Year-round when accessible; fees
collected Memorial Day weekend–
Labor Day only

SITES: 7

EACH SITE: Picnic table, fire grate

ASSIGNMENT: First come, first served;
no reservations

REGISTRATION: On-site self-registration

FACILITIES: Hand-pump well, vault toilets

PARKING: At campsites

FEE: $10

ELEVATION: 5,300'

RESTRICTIONS:

Pets: On leash only

Fires: In fire rings only

Alcohol: Permitted

Vehicles: 35-foot length limit

Other: 16-day stay limit; bear-country
food-storage precautions recommended;
pack in, pack out

Sites 1–4 also border the cold-running creek, where anglers catch brook trout and waders cool off on hot afternoons. The remaining sites, 6 and 7, are well separated from each other and everyone else. Every site here is good, with plenty of room to pitch a tent and spread out.

Other base camp options here include the dispersed campsite on the left just before you get to the campground and Crazy Creek Campground (off the East Fork Road west of Sula). Crazy Creek does have more of a wilderness feel than Martin Creek, but it's adjacent to an equestrian trailhead, and you may have trouble finding a level spot to pitch a tent. Overall, it's a good alternative and still close to hiking opportunities.

Forest Road 5765 leads to the McCart Lookout Trail. The 5.5-mile drive to the trailhead is on a rough but beautiful mountain road that is easily passable in dry conditions. Be cautious if it is wet, since the road may be slick, especially on the downhill trip. From the trailhead, it's a 1.5-mile hike to a lookout that has been retired from active fire use and is now available for rent. McCart has been restored to reflect a 1940s lookout, giving visitors a chance to experience what the original structure looked like. It is listed on the National Register of Historic Places and sits on the edge of the Anaconda-Pintlar Wilderness, offering beautiful views of the Pintlar Mountains to the east and the Bitterroot Mountains to the west.

The Chain-of-Lakes trailhead lies past the ranger station, about 2.5 miles up FR 726. From here you can take a fairly strenuous, 13-mile out-and-back trail that leads to Hope, Faith, and Charity Lakes. The trailhead for Moose Creek Trail #168 is about 2 miles past the campground on FR 432. The first few miles of this trail follow the creek as it winds along the canyon.

Martin Creek Campground

GETTING THERE

From Sula, take County Road 101 east 16 miles to FR 726. Turn left to the campground.

GPS COORDINATES: N45° 55.922' W113° 43.345'

46

⛺ May Creek Campground

Beauty: ★★★★ / Privacy: ★★★★ / Quiet: ★★★★ / Spaciousness: ★★★ / Security: ★★★★ /
Cleanliness: ★★★★

If you've simply looking for the peace afforded so splendidly throughout the Big Hole, this campground may be all you need.

The peaceful, beautiful landscapes reached from the campground in any direction hardly resemble a war zone. Meadows, wildflowers, dense forest, rivers, and creeks, all bedecked by the backdrop of the Beaverhead and Pioneer Mountains, is home to a vast array of wildlife without showing a hint of discord. Unfortunately, however, human blood was indeed spilled near here when in 1877 the Nez Perce took up arms rather than agreeing to internment on a reservation located on a fragment of their traditional homeland. Several lives were lost on both sides of the Nez Perce War of 1877, a tragedy that climaxed over four battles, one of which occurred within the Big Hole Basin. The remaining Nez Perce reluctantly moved to the reservation after suffering a closing blow in the final battle near the Canada border, just 40 miles from freedom. Those who lost their lives are honored just 8 miles from the campground at the Big Hole National Battlefield.

The visitor center, which overlooks the actual battlefield, shelters artifacts and photographs from the battle. Video programs, self-guided trails, and ranger-led programs will keep you busy during your visit, revealing a multitude of details regarding the conflict and the plight of the Nez Perce. All this is eye-opening and definitely worth the visit.

If a war story is not your thing and you are simply looking for the peace afforded so splendidly throughout the valley, the campground may be all you need. The sites are comfortable and well spaced on comparatively flat ground.

Another way to enjoy the peace is go fishing. May Creek flows near the west side of the campground through pine forest, where the scrappy brookies and rainbow trout just

A typical campsite at May Creek Campground provides the basics and access to fishing, hiking, historical landscapes, and peaceful interaction with nature.

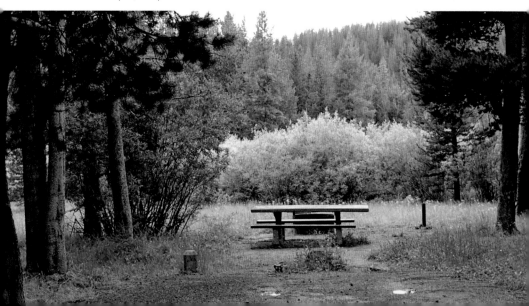

KEY INFORMATION

ADDRESS: MT 43, Wisdom, MT 59761

CONTACT: 406-689-3243,
www.fs.usda.gov/bdnf

OPERATED BY: Beaverhead-Deerlodge
National Forest, Wisdom Ranger District

OPEN: May–October or November; water
available through September only

SITES: 21

EACH SITE: Picnic table, fire ring

ASSIGNMENT: First come, first served;
no reservations

REGISTRATION: On-site self-registration

FACILITIES: Hand-pump well, vault toilets

PARKING: At campsites

FEE: $7

ELEVATION: 6,300′

RESTRICTIONS:

Pets: On leash only

Fires: In fire rings only

Alcohol: Permitted

Vehicles: 30-foot length limit

Other: 16-day stay limit; bear-country
food storage restrictions; pack in,
pack out

might be hungry when you stroll over. For larger fare, the Blue Ribbon fishery of the Big Hole River is where larger trout fight for keeps, and you might even entice a fluvial Arctic grayling. Travel 17 miles back to the town of Wisdom on US 43 and visit the fishing access sites of Fishtrap Creek and Sportsman's Park, both located north of Wisdom.

Moose, elk, and deer are frequently seen in the open near the campground, along the roads, and on hikes, where you could also see hawks, kestrels, falcons, golden eagles, coyotes, and maybe a bear. The area is an elk-calving area so, depending on the timing of your visit, you could encounter a herd of elk with young'uns.

The entire valley is a popular place to view wildlife, but your chances increase while hiking

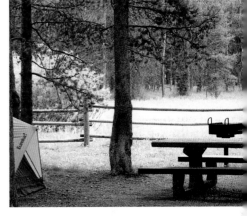

You are blessedly on your own at May Creek Campground—but keep a watchful eye out for wildlife!

the trails that branch out from and near the campground. From the campground the May Creek Trail #103 follows the creek over easy terrain, bypassing the May Creek Cabin at just under the 2-mile mark. You can rest and turn around here or explore beyond the cabin. Or you can keep going for a bigger out-and-back adventure. About 7 miles up the drainage the trail eventually intercepts the Continental Divide Trail along Anderson Mountain Road (Forest Road 081).

If your visit of the historic May Creek Cabin struck your fancy, the cabin can be rented at recreation.gov for $25 a night. The cabin was constructed in the 1920s to provide housing for forest workers who kept busy building trail, fighting fires, and cutting timber. Staying at the cabin is a do-it-yourself option with no water, electricity, or garbage service, although it is provisioned for four people with firewood, a wood-burning stove, two bunk beds, a table, benches, and a propane stove for cooking, but no propane. You must bring in your own propane canisters. Pack out what you pack in.

Soakers can delight in the fact the campground is within an easy drive of two natural, geothermally heated hot springs. The closest is Jackson Hot Springs, located 18 miles south of Wisdom on MT 278. The other, more rustic, mineral pool is Elkhorn Hot Springs, located nearly an hour from Wisdom. To soak at Elkhorn, travel about 36 miles south on MT 278 and turn left on Polaris Road/Pioneer Mountains Scenic Byway, and drive north for 15 miles to the hot springs. Good eats are available in the restaurants at both of these fun hot spring retreats.

May Creek Campground

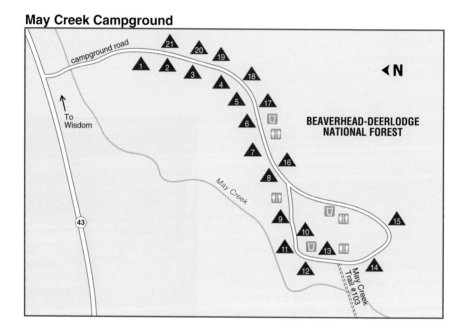

GETTING THERE

From Wisdom, take US 43 west for 17 miles to the campground entrance, on the left.

GPS COORDINATES: N45° 39.038' W113° 46.981'

47

Miner Lake Campground

Beauty: ★★★★ / Privacy: ★★★★ / Quiet: ★★★ / Spaciousness: ★★★★ / Security: ★★★ /
Cleanliness: ★★★★

A pair of mountain lakes offers a peaceful place to relax and set up a hiking base camp.

With a scenic drive in and access to numerous hiking trails, this pair of mountain lakes is an ideal choice if you seek a peaceful place to relax and set up a hiking base camp. The campground sits on the larger of the Lower Miner Lakes and offers views of the surrounding Beaverhead Mountains. There are two choices for camping, and the better one is the designated campground area on the main body of the lake. Sites are spacious, with plenty of trees, but there are enough openings that they are sunlit at least part of the day. Sites 12, 14, and 15 are the best overall, with lake views and plenty of room to spread out. Located next to the day-use area, Site 11 is just as roomy with good views, but depending on the group, daytime noise may be too much for those who stay close to camp.

Campsites along the entrance road, especially sites 1–5, overlook a lily pad–filled section of the lakes. These sites are smaller and less private, but the bugs aren't as bad as you might expect. Nighttime temperatures at this altitude, even in the middle of summer, can get mighty cold. You could awaken to snow and then face temperatures in the 80s by midafternoon; be sure to pack accordingly.

A restriction on gas-powered motors makes Miner Lake a perfect place for canoeing. The clear green water is chillier than it looks, so your swimming time may be limited. Fishing for rainbow and Yellowstone cutthroat trout, burbot, or Arctic grayling can be an excellent way to begin or end the day.

Launch a new adventure or get into some great fishing from a canoe or kayak at Miner Lake.

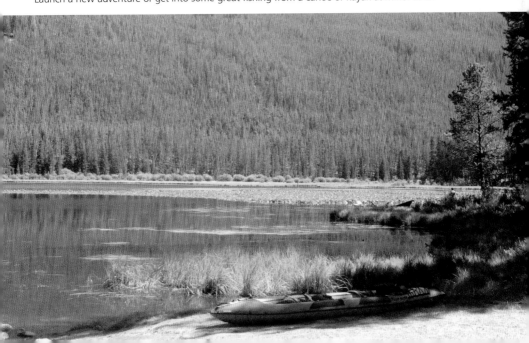

KEY INFORMATION

ADDRESS: Miner Lake Road
(Forest Road 182), Jackson, MT 59736

CONTACT: 406-689-3243,
www.fs.usda.gov/bdnf

OPERATED BY: Beaverhead-Deerlodge
National Forest, Wisdom Ranger District

OPEN: Generally accessible June–September,
depending on snow; full services available
July and August only

SITES: 18

EACH SITE: Picnic table, fire grate

ASSIGNMENT: First come, first served;
no reservations

REGISTRATION: On-site self-registration

FACILITIES: Hand-pump well, vault toilets,
carry-in boat launch

PARKING: At campsites

FEE: $7

ELEVATION: 7,000'

RESTRICTIONS:

Pets: On leash only

Fires: In fire rings only

Alcohol: Permitted

Vehicles: 20-foot length limit

Other: 16-day stay limit; bear-country
food storage restrictions; pack in,
pack out; nonmotorized boats only

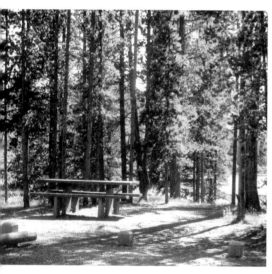

Several campsites at Miner Lake Campground are within easy reach of the lake.

Because designated travel routes in the immediate area are open to motorized use, note that you may encounter four-wheelers or motorcycles. Travel restrictions begin 2 miles down the road, where a gate marks the trailhead and the end of the road for vehicles. The road from the campground to the trailhead is unmaintained and rough.

Hikes from this trailhead run along the eastern slope of the Continental Divide and are considered part of the Continental Divide Trail. The first mile or so is a slow uphill to a fork where you can go left and hike another 2 miles to Upper Miner Lake. Otherwise, 2 miles on the right fork take you to Rock Island Lakes Trail #54, followed by a short, steep climb to Little Lake Trail #87. If you're not dizzy from the altitude, take another steep climb to the top of the Divide and a view to the east of Homer Youngs Peak. At 10,621 feet, it's one of the tallest peaks in the West Big Hole Mountains.

This is also Nez Perce (Ne-Me-Poo) Trail country. During the summer of 1877, Chief Joseph trekked 1,100 miles over three and a half months with a group made up mainly of women, children, the sick, and the elderly. This hardy band of 750 fought over 20 battles against 2,000 troops on their doomed flight toward Canada and freedom. On August 9, the group was ambushed in a battle where both sides suffered severe casualties. The Big Hole National Battlefield outside Wisdom provides interpretive programs and access to the battlefield itself. The Nez Perce National Historic Trail runs along MT 278 in this area, and additional information is available at the Battlefield visitor center.

It's only 10 miles to the tiny town of Jackson (population 50), where everyone's water comes preheated to about 135 degrees from its hot-springs source. In 1806, William Clark dutifully recorded the facts: "This Spring contains a very considerable quantity of water, and actually blubbers with heat for 20 paces below where it rises. It has every appearance of boiling, too hot for a man to endure his hand in it 3 seconds." He then moved on to experimentation by using the springs to cook wild game. "The [piece of meat] about the Size of my 2 fingers Cooked dun in 25 minutes the other much thicker was 32 minits before it became Sufficiently dun." Today's visitors use the water for soaking and relaxing at Jackson Hot Springs and have their meals at the restaurant cooked on the stove.

As you drive throughout the Big Hole Valley, you may see large wooden contraptions that look a little like catapults sitting in the middle of fields. These are called beaver slides and were invented by two local ranchers in 1910 to help them stack hay. Not much has changed over the past century in this "Land of 10,000 Haystacks," and you'll still see the slides being used during haying season.

Miner Lake Campground

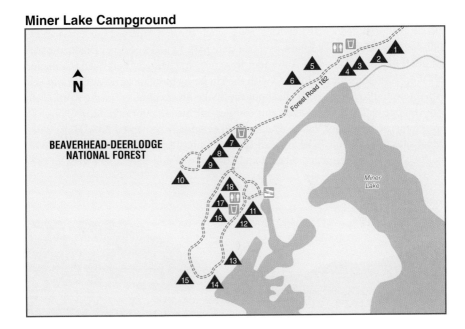

GETTING THERE

From Jackson, take MT 278 south for 0.5 miles to CR 182 (Miner Lake Road). Turn right and go 10 miles west to the campground. (After 7 miles, the road becomes Forest Service Road 182 and narrows.)

GPS COORDINATES: N45° 19.462' W113° 34.687'

48

⛺ Reservoir Lake Campground

Beauty: ★★★★★ / Privacy: ★★★★ / Quiet: ★★★ / Spaciousness: ★★★★★ / Security: ★★★★ /
Cleanliness: ★★★★★

Your campsite will be only 3 miles as the crow flies from the Idaho–Montana border and the Continental Divide Trail.

Set on a 45-acre lake in a narrow slice of the Beaverhead-Deerlodge National Forest, this campground is a quiet respite after a beautiful, albeit bumpy, 60-mile drive from Dillon. On the drive, you'll pass through sagebrush plains and grasslands and may begin to doubt that there is a forest at the end of the road, but the Beaverhead Mountains loom ahead of you, and your campsite will be only 3 miles as the crow flies from the Idaho–Montana border and the Continental Divide Trail. The access road, part of the designated Nez Perce National Historic Trail, follows a portion of the route used by Chief Joseph as he valiantly attempted to lead the Nez Perce across the Canadian border to safety.

The Beaverhead portion of the forest and the mountain range are named after a rock formation near Dillon that the Shoshone thought resembled the head of a swimming beaver. A significant landmark recognized by Sacagawea when she accompanied the Lewis and Clark Expedition, Beaverhead Rock is now part of a state park 13 miles north of Dillon, on MT 41.

Another explorer, Canadian Alexander Ross, was in charge of Fort Walla Walla for the North West Company until it merged with the Hudson's Bay Company, and he was sent on an expedition to provide more detail about the Snake River country. During April, October, and November of 1824, he traveled and camped in this area until crossing Gibbon's Pass and reaching the Bitterroot Valley, which would eventually be named Ross' Hole.

Most sites at Reservoir Lake are well spaced. Only sites 8 and 11, on the inside of one of the loop roads, feel crowded. Sites 9 and 10 are large and have a nice view of the lake

Reservoir Lake

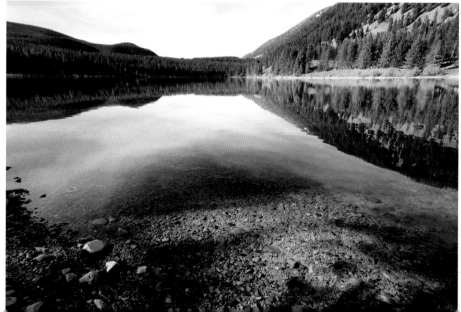

photo: D. Tate/flickr.com/photos/18toks

KEY INFORMATION

ADDRESS: Bloody Dick Road
(Forest Road 181), Dillon, MT 59725

CONTACT: 406-683-3900,
www.fs.usda.gov/bdnf

OPERATED BY: Beaverhead-Deerlodge
National Forest, Dillon Ranger District

OPEN: Year-round when accessible; fees and
water mid-June–mid-September only

SITES: 15

EACH SITE: Picnic table, fire ring

ASSIGNMENT: First come, first served;
no reservations

REGISTRATION: On-site self-registration

FACILITIES: Water spigot, vault toilets,
boat launch

PARKING: At campsites

FEE: $8, $2/additional vehicle

ELEVATION: 7,065'

RESTRICTIONS:

Pets: On leash only

Fires: In fire rings only

Alcohol: Permitted

Vehicles: 16-foot length limit

Other: 16-day stay limit; bear-country food
storage restrictions; pack in, pack-out

through the trees. Site 15, roomy as well, is set on a high spot overlooking the lily pads on the southwestern end of the lake. This site is in the open and perfect for those seeking the early morning sun and clear views of the night sky. Sites 16 and 17 sit by themselves on a short spur road. There is ample space between these and sites 12 and 13, on the inside of the second loop road. Shy away from site 7—it has a good view but is near the outhouse and day-use parking lot.

Don't leave the canoe behind when visiting this campground. You will probably want to paddle the lake's shimmering, clear water. Swimming sessions may be short, as the water remains cold well into summer, although the chilly temperature is not much of a deterrent for swimmers young and old. Fishing is for brook trout and can be just as successful from the shore as from a boat.

A motor restriction on the lake helps keep things quiet, but you will encounter motorized vehicles like ATVs and motorbikes in the surrounding area, since some forest roads are open to motorized use. Notices requesting riders to push their machines out of the campground before starting them up are posted, but this rarely happens. Thankfully, most drivers are respectful and travel at slow speeds.

Bloody Dick Creek runs to the west of the lake and offers fishing for mountain whitefish and brook and rainbow trout. Both the creek and nearby Bloody Dick Peak (9,817') were named for an early English settler named Richards who liberally sprinkled his conversation with the very British adjective *bloody*. About a half mile from the campground is another namesake for Mr. Richards: Bloody Dick Cabin. This one-room cabin can be reserved at recreation.gov for those who might opt for a bunk bed and a roof.

A variety of trails beckons hikers and bikers alike. Eunice Creek Trail #157 provides access to the Continental Divide Trail, and Trail #77 runs north on a ridge above the creek. A shorter but still steep trail heads northeast from the campground to Selway Mountain, where the views across the Divide are dramatic.

Reservoir Lake Campground

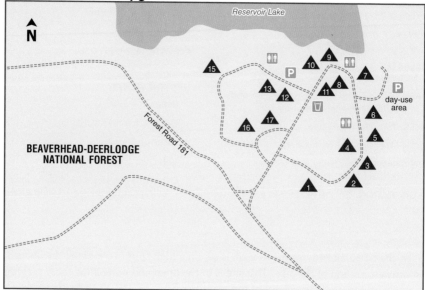

GETTING THERE

From Dillon, take I-15 south for 19 miles to Exit 44, and take MT 324 west for 17 miles to Forest Road 181. Turn right and go 18 miles to the campground.

GPS COORDINATES: N45° 7.306' W113° 27.245'

49

Twin Lakes Campground

Beauty: ★★★★★ / Privacy: ★★★★ / Quiet: ★★★★ / Spaciousness: ★★★★ / Security: ★★★★ / Cleanliness: ★★★★

If you're lucky, creek crossings may reveal a great blue heron looking for lunch.

Here in the Big Hole River valley, famous as "The Land of 10,000 Haystacks," the setting sun casts its glow on endless stretches of ranchland broken only by cottonwoods lining the riverbanks and haystacks set against a glorious mountain backdrop. Early settlers used the term "Big Hole" for any wide mountain valley, and here the name stuck. It's easy to understand why the people who make this valley their home are willing to put in the long hours to make a living here. It is a land of cattle and sagebrush, a history filled with stories of gold, and fishing on one of the nation's most famous trout streams in a landscape that played an integral part in the Nez Perce tribe's 1877 flight to Canada.

Chief Joseph and the Nez Perce tribe broke camp after the Battle of the Big Hole and headed south on August 10, 1877. This hardy group would travel the length of the Bitterroot Mountains, across Bannack Pass, and well into Idaho over the next five days. Think about it: this wasn't just a group of young warriors; there were plenty of women and children, too. They had been traveling for weeks, had just fought one battle, and would walk nearly 150 miles as the crow flies across the steep mountains you see around you, arriving at the site of the Birch Creek Affair on August 15. Makes any hiking we do seem pretty simple, doesn't it?

The drive to Twin Lakes is a journey where you should take your time, not only because the road is rough but also because there is no reason to rush. The scenery is just too beautiful, and when you slow down you can encounter all kinds of delights. Watch for deer—you're sure to see some. Keep an eye out for hawks and golden eagles perched in snags or soaring high above, and if you're lucky, creek crossings may reveal a great blue heron looking for lunch.

All campsites are just a short walk from the lakeshore.

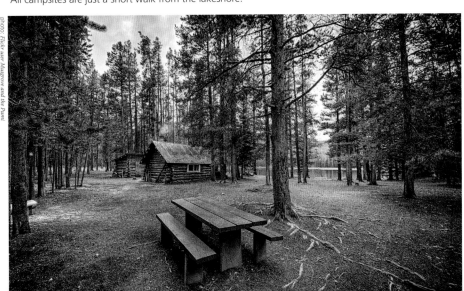

KEY INFORMATION

ADDRESS: Forest Road 183, Wisdom, MT 59761

CONTACT: 406-689-3243, www.fs.usda.gov/bdnf

OPERATED BY: Beaverhead-Deerlodge National Forest, Wisdom Ranger District

OPEN: Late June–October, weather permitting; water available through Labor Day only

SITES: 17

EACH SITE: Picnic table, fire ring

ASSIGNMENT: First come, first served; no reservations

REGISTRATION: On-site self-registration

FACILITIES: Hand-pump well, vault toilets, carry-in boat launch

PARKING: At campsites

FEE: $7

ELEVATION: 7,200'

RESTRICTIONS:

Pets: On leash only

Fires: In fire rings only

Alcohol: Permitted

Vehicles: 25-foot length limit

Other: 16-day stay limit; bear-country food storage restrictions; pack in, pack out; nonmotorized boats only

Sites at Twin Lakes are nicely spaced; the first three are located just beyond the turnoff from Forest Road 183. Sites 4–10 are great locations near the lakeshore, allowing unimpeded access and offering a thick cover of pines for shade. Sites 12–17 are on the inside of the loop created by the main road and the campground road, and while they are great sites with good views of the lake, they are not as private as the others, and road noise and dust may be bothersome.

Twin Lakes is actually a single body of water along Big Lake Creek, and this 84-acre lake is an excellent place to use a canoe or kayak to explore or to fish for grayling and brook, rainbow, or lake trout. Those without boats can easily spend an entire day wading, skipping rocks, fishing from shore, and even swimming in the heat of the day. Nighttime temperatures at this altitude, even in the middle of summer, can reach freezing. You could awaken to snow and then face high temperatures by midafternoon.

Another option for anglers is to head for the west end of the lake. The creek here is particularly good with a fly rod, lightweight tippet, and a size-22 Griffith's Gnat employed upstream of a pool or along a bank undercut.

This is also an excellent location if you want to try a section of the Continental Divide Trail. Twin Lakes Trail #467 begins at the entrance to the campground and can be used as an easy 4-mile out-and-back hike, or you can keep going another 0.75 mile along pioneered routes to the Divide. To the south is Slag-a-melt Creek, and to the north is Jumbo Mountain.

Originally called Crossings and then Noyes, the town of Wisdom is still little more than a crossroads, but it's the closest town to Twin Lakes. A stop for a cold drink and a burger will introduce you to some of the finest and friendliest folks around, and the conversation will range from the weather to politics to local gossip.

Twin Lakes Campground

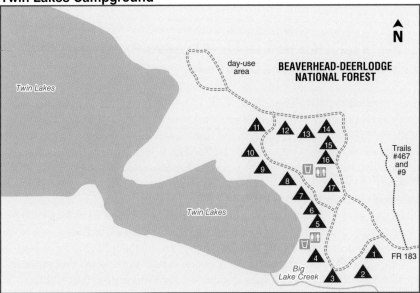

GETTING THERE

From Wisdom, take MT 278 south for 7 miles to CR 1290. Turn right and go 8 miles west to FR 945. Turn left and go 5 miles south to FR 183. Turn right and go 5 miles southwest to the campground.

GPS COORDINATES: N45° 24.662' W113° 41.271'

50

Three Frogs Campground

Beauty: ★★★★ / Privacy: ★★★ / Quiet: ★★★ / Spaciousness: ★★★★ / Security: ★★★★★ /
Cleanliness: ★★★★★

This camp is set within thick stands of Douglas-fir and lodgepole pine, with views of El Capitan and Como Peaks.

This newly reconstructed campground, with 16 small-trailer sites and 4 walk-in sites, is definitely as tent friendly as its predecessor, the Upper Como Lake Campground.

With the 9,000-foot-plus El Capitan and Como Peaks reflecting in the water and access to the recreational facilities on Lake Como all within walking distance, this is a busy location, so arriving here midweek may be your best bet for securing a choice spot. Set among thick stands of lodgepole pine and fir, sites here are spacious and level, even though the campground road climbs a bit as you make your way along the one-way loop road.

There's no water within the interior of the campground, so be sure to look for the available spigots off to the right just before the fee sign at the trailhead near site 1, or you can fill up in the lower campground. Even though campers are encouraged to practice bear-aware food-storage precautions, you may still encounter a bear in the area. Precautionary and safety information is posted at the fee station, and the campground host will know about the latest sightings.

Cooling off in the lake is a popular pastime, and the beach and roped-off swimming area can get crowded on warm summer weekends, so stake out your spot early. Motorboats and water-skiers dominate on weekends, but even then there are still quiet spots for canoes. Fishing the lake is also popular, and many anglers will try their luck at landing a rainbow trout, kokanee, Westslope cutthroat trout, or mountain whitefish.

This campground offers two great trails to explore if you're looking for a short morning hike before everyone else gets up. One is above the campground, and the other circles the pond. For a longer hike, the 7-mile Lake Como National Recreational Loop Trail starts from the trailhead near site 1 and begins with a 0.25-mile disabled-accessible surface. The section along the north shore (Trail #502) is for foot and bicycle travel only

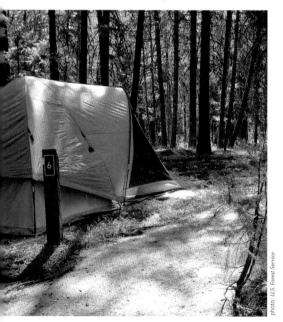

Three Frogs is a popular campground, so try to arrive midweek to secure a good site.

photo: U.S. Forest Service

KEY INFORMATION

ADDRESS: Lake Como Road, Darby, MT 59829

CONTACT: 406-821-3913, www.fs.usda.gov /bitterroot

OPERATED BY: Bitterroot National Forest, Darby Ranger District

OPEN: Mid-May–September; limited services after Labor Day

SITES: 20

EACH SITE: Picnic table, fire grate

ASSIGNMENT: First come, first served; no reservations

REGISTRATION: On-site self-registration

FACILITIES: Water spigot, vault toilets, beach, boat launch

PARKING: At campsites

FEE: $8

ELEVATION: 4,500'

RESTRICTIONS:

Pets: On leash only

Fires: In fire rings only

Alcohol: Permitted

Vehicles: 30-foot length limit

Other: 16-day stay limit; bear-country food-storage precautions recommended

---

and offers wildflower meadows and views of the Como Peaks, while the southern half of the loop (Trail #580) is also open to horses, is not as scenic, and ends near the beach area. Both trails stay close to the water and provide plenty of bird-watching opportunities.

From the campground it's about 3.5 miles to the west end of the lake and the waterfall. There you can take Trail #580 to the west, instead of continuing around the lake, and travel a route along Rock Creek through a densely forested, steep canyon. The mile from the waterfall and pack bridge traverses an area recovering from the 1988 fire, but once hikers enter the Selway-Bitterroot Wilderness, the forest becomes green again. This trail is heavily used by pack horses, but for those up to a challenge, offshoots from the rushing Rock Creek waters offer crossings that range from easy to treacherous. Plan to head back to the campground when you reach a crossing that is beyond your skill level. Successfully fording the creek once may provide an adrenaline rush, but remember you'll have to approach it again, and you'll be more tired and prone to injury. Always err on the side of caution—it doesn't make you a wimp, and it just might keep you in one piece instead of ruining a great vacation.

The entire Lake Como area has always been a significant wildlife corridor, and all hiking trails provide opportunities to observe a variety of species. Large populations of elk, moose, and white-tailed deer exist, but when there is heavy trail use, they'll be scarce.

Located in Darby is the historic Darby Ranger Station Visitor Center and Museum. Open daily (except Sundays) May–October, 8:30 a.m.–4:30 p.m., it provides informative displays about Depression-era Civilian Conservation Corps and U.S. Forest Service history. The helpful staff is ready and willing to answer questions and distribute information about hiking trails, recreation, and road conditions.

Three Frogs Campground

GETTING THERE

From Darby, take US 93 north for 4 miles. Turn left on County Road 82 and go 4 miles west to the campground.

From Hamilton, take US 93 south for 12 miles. Turn right on CR 82 and go 4 miles west to the campground.

GPS COORDINATES: N46° 3.985' W114° 14.936'

APPENDIX A:

CAMPING-EQUIPMENT CHECKLIST

Camping is more fun when you can enjoy it at a moment's notice. You never know when the opportunity may arise to head for the hills, and when it does, wouldn't it be nice to be able to pack your car with prepacked boxes of essentials that were carefully cleaned, resupplied, and stored after your last trip? It's a nice fantasy isn't it? Unfortunately, it's one we've never actually experienced, but we do keep trying.

COOKING/KITCHEN
(Packed in a plastic box)
Bowls
Can opener
Cook pots with lids
Cooler
Dishcloth and towel
Dishpan
Dry-food box
Dutch oven and fire pan
5-gallon water jug
Flatwear
Frying pan
Insulated plastic mugs
Large serving spoon
Lighter or matches
Paper towels
Plates
Pocketknife
Rain tarp or dining fly
Sharp knife
Spatula
Spices, salt, pepper
Stove and fuel
Strainer
Tablecloth
Tinfoil
Trash bags
Wooden spoon

SLEEPING QUARTERS
Ground cloth
Pillow
Sleeping bag
Sleeping pad
Tent and rainfly

MISCELLANEOUS
Candles
Day pack
Extra batteries
Firewood
First aid kit
Flashlight
Folding camp chair
Lantern
Maps
Premoistened towels
Resealable plastic bags
Saw/ax
Toilet paper
Water bottles

OPTIONAL
Binoculars
Books
Camera
Cards and games
Field guides
Fishing rod
Frisbee

APPENDIX B:

SOURCES OF INFORMATION

BEAVERHEAD-DEERLODGE NATIONAL FOREST

420 Barrett St.
Dillon, MT 59725
406-683-3900, 406-683-3913
(24-hour recorded information)
www.fs.usda.gov/bdnf

BITTERROOT NATIONAL FOREST

1801 N. First St.
Hamilton, MT 59840
406-363-7100
www.fs.usda.gov/bitterroot

BUREAU OF LAND MANAGEMENT

Montana/Dakotas State Office
5001 Southgate Drive
Billings, MT 59101
406-896-5000
blm.gov/mt/st/en.html

BUREAU OF RECLAMATION

Montana Area Office
406-247-7300
usbr.gov/gp/mtao

CUSTER GALLATIN NATIONAL FOREST

10 E. Babcock Ave.
Bozeman, MT 59771
406-587-6701
www.fs.usda.gov/custergallatin

FLATHEAD NATIONAL FOREST

650 Wolfpack Way
Kalispell, MT 59901
406-758-5208
www.fs.usda.gov/flathead

GLACIER NATIONAL PARK

Park Headquarters
PO Box 128/64 Grinnell Drive
West Glacier, MT 59936
406-888-7800
nps.gov/glac

HELENA–LEWIS AND CLARK NATIONAL FOREST

2880 Skyway Drive
Helena, MT 59602
406-449-5201
www.fs.usda.gov/hlcnf, www.fs.usda.gov/helena

KOOTENAI NATIONAL FOREST

31374 US 2
Libby, MT 59923
406-293-6211
www.fs.usda.gov/kootenai

LOLO NATIONAL FOREST

24 Fort Missoula Road
Missoula, MT 59804
406-329-3750
www.fs.usda.gov/lolo

MONTANA FISH, WILDLIFE & PARKS

1420 E. Sixth Ave.
Helena, MT 59620
406-444-2535
Relay 711 or 800-253-4091 (TDD)
fwp.mt.gov

MONTANA DEPARTMENT OF NATURAL RESOURCES & CONSERVATION

1625 11th Ave.
Helena, MT 59601
406-444-2074
dnrc.mt.gov

MONTANA OFFICE OF TOURISM

301 S. Park Ave.
Helena, MT 59620
406-841-2870, 800-847-4868
visitmt.com

MONTANA WILDERNESS ASSOCIATION

80 S. Warren St.
Helena, MT 59601
406-443-7350
wildmontana.org

U.S. ARMY CORPS OF ENGINEERS
Fort Peck Dam & Lake
406-526-3411
tinyurl.com/acefortpeck

**U.S. FOREST SERVICE,
NORTHERN REGION**

Federal Building
PO Box 7669/200 E. Broadway
Missoula, MT 59807
406-329-3511
www.fs.usda.gov/r1

YELLOWSTONE NATIONAL PARK
Yellowstone National Park, WY 82190
307-344-7381, 307-344-2386 (TTY)
nps.gov/yell

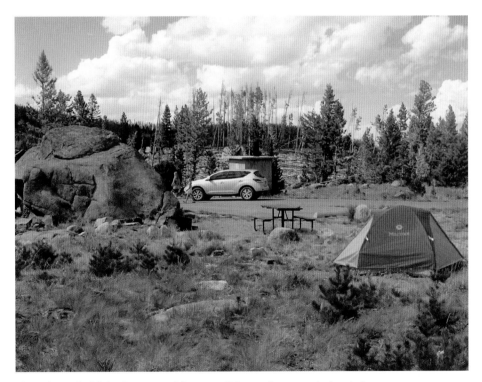

Campsites at Park Lake Campground *(see page 67)* range from open to forested.

INDEX

Page references followed by *m* indicate a map.

A. B. Guthrie Trail, 53
Absaroka-Beartooth Wilderness, 116
Adventure Medical, 5
Albro Lake Trail #333, 113
alcohol restrictions. *See specific campground*
American Indians. *See* Native Americans
Anaconda (Montana), 147–148
animals. *See* wildlife
Arapooish, Chief, 90

Atwater Carey, 5

Babcock Mountain, 142
Bad Medicine Campground, 12–14*m*
Bangtail Divide Trail #504, 95
Bannack ghost town ("toughest town in the West"), 134–135
Bannack State Park Campground, 134–136*m*
Basin Lakes National Recreation Trail #6, 116
Bass Creek, 137
Bass Creek Recreation Area, 137–139*m*
Bass Creek Scenic Overlook, 137
Bass Creek Trail #4, 138
Bass Lake, 138
bathing, 10
bathroom planning, 8–9
Battle Ridge Campground, 94–96*m*
Bear Creek Saloon and Steakhouse, 117
Bear Paw Battlefield (Nez Perce National Historical Park), 77, 82
bears *See also specific campground*
    "bear aware" behavior, 81
    precautions for avoiding, 6
    protecting your site from, 9
Bear Paw Mountains, 77
beauty rating, 1, 2
Beaver Creek, 77–79*m*
Beaver Creek Campground, 97–99*m*
Beaver Creek County Park Campgrounds, 77–79*m*
Beaverhead-Deerlodge National Forest
    Lost Creek State Park Campground adjacent to, 146–148*m*
    Reservoir Lake Campground in the, 158–160*m*
Beaverhead Mountains, 158

Bell Lake Trail #305, 113
Belt Creek, 61
Big Arm Unit–Flathead Lake State Park Campground, 15–17*m*
Big Creek, 18–20*m*
Big Creek Campground, 18–20*m*
Big George Gulch Trail #251, 57
Big Hole National Battlefield, 152, 156–157, 161
Big Hole River, 153
Big Hole Valley ("Land of 10,000 Haystacks"), 157, 161
Big Lake Creek, 162
Big Snowy Mountains, 83
Big Therriault Lake Campground, 21–23*m*
Big Therriault Lake, 22, 23*m*
Big Timber Creek Trail #119, 107
Big Timber Falls (or Halfmoon Falls), 107
Big Timber Peak, 107
bighorn sheep. *See* Rocky Mountain bighorn
bird-watching. *See specific campground*
Black Pyramid Mountain, 105
Blackfeet Indians
    Sun River, named Medicine River by, 55
    Thain Creek, named *Espi-toh-tok* by, 70
Blackfoot Meadow, 59
Blackfoot Meadow Trail #329, 59
Blackfoot River, 36
Blackmore Trail #423, 109
Blacktail Creek Trail #223, 56
Bloody Dick Cabin, 159
Bloody Dick Creek, 159
Bloody Dick Peak, 159
Blossom Lake Trail #404, 49
Blue Creek Trail #425, 144
Blue Lake, 107
Blue Ribbon fishery (Big Hole River), 153
Bluebird Lake, 22
Bob Marshall Wilderness Area ("The Bob"), 56, 73, 74
Bob Marshall Wilderness Complex, 73
Boulder Creek, 144
Boulder Mountains, 67
Bozeman Pass, 94

Bridger Bowl Ski Area, 94
Briggs Creek Trail #431, 71
Brown's Lake Trail #2, 144
"Buffalo Soldiers" (10th Cavalry), 77
Bull River Guard Station (1908), 13
Bullhead Lodge, 27

Cabinet Mountain Wilderness, 12–14*m*
Camp Creek Campground, 80–82*m*
campsites
    advance preparation
        picking your camping buddies, 8
        reservations, 8
    courtesy
        Leave No Trace practices, 10, 144
        to other campers, 10
    food preparation
        bringing in supplies, 9
        cleaning and bear protection, 9, 81
        fire rings and restrictions, 9–10
        washing dishes/laundry/bathing, 10
    setting up
        bathroom planning, 8–9
        check in, pay fee, mark site, 8
        don't tie things to trees, 8
        tents, 8
campground information
    additional sources of, 168–169
    campground profile, 3
    GPS entrance coordinates, 3
    layout maps, 3
    rating system, 1–2
camping tips
    camping-equipment checklist, 167
    plan ahead, 7
    reserve site in advance, 8
    setting up your site, 8–10
    while traveling, 7
Carbon County Museum, 116
Cave Mountain Campground, 52–54*m*
cell phone coverage, 4
Chain-of-Lakes Trail, 150
Charles M. Russell National Wildlife Refuge, 81
Charles Waters Campground, 137–139*m*
Charter Oak Mine, 58
Chippewa Cree tribe Rocky Boy's Reservation, 77,
    78–79
Civilian Conservation Corps, 59, 165
Clark Fork River, 48–50*m*
Clark, William, 147, 157
Clary Coulee Trail #177, 52
cleanliness rating, 1, 2
Clearwater Canoe Trail, 37
Clearwater Chain-of-Lakes driving tour, 38
Clearwater River, 36

Cliff Lake, 127–129*m*
clotheslines, 8
clothing recommendations, 8
Coal Miner's Park, 116
Conical Peak, 107
Continental Divide Trail
    Miner Lake Campground, 156
    Reservoir Lake Campground, 158, 159
    Twin Lakes Campground, 162
Cooke City (Montana), 115
copper mining, 147
courtesy
    Leave No Trace practices, 10, 144
    to other campers, 10
    protection practices, 9–10
Cramton, Louis C., 45
Crazy Creek Campground, 150
Crazy Mountains (*Awaxaawippiia*), 106
Crazy Peak, 107, 108
Crow Indians
    Chief Arapooish and Chief Plenty Coups
        leaders of, 90
    Crazy Mountains named *Awaxaawippiia* by
        the, 106
Crystal Cascades Trail #445, 84
Crystal Lake, 83, 84, 85*m*
Crystal Lake Campground, 83–85*m*
Crystal Park, 144
Curry, Kid, 80
Cut Bank Campground, 24–26*m*
Cut Bank Creek, 25

Dalles Campground, 140–142*m*
Darby Ranger Station Visitor Center and Museum,
    165
Deer Creek Trail #453, 71
DEET, 7
Demers Ridge Trail, 19
DeSmet, Father Pierre, 138
dinosaur fossils. *See* fossils
Dirty Shame Saloon, 39
Discovery Center (Apgar, Montana), 29
dish washing tips, 10
Double Falls, 74
dress recommendations, 8

Eastern Montana
    Beaver Creek County Park Campgrounds, 77–79*m*
    Camp Creek Campground, 80–82*m*
    Crystal Lake Campground, 83–85*m*
    Makoshika State Park Campground, 86–89*m*
    Sage Creek Campground, 90–92*m*
Egg Mountain, 54
Elkhorn Hot Springs, 143, 144, 154
Eunice Creek Trail #157, 159

Face of the Mountain trailhead and Trail #7, 116
Fairmont Hot Springs (resort), 148
Fairy Lake, 95
Fairy Lake Campground, 95
Falls Creek, 100
Falls Creek Campground, 100–102m
fees See also specific campground
  checking in and paying the campground, 8
  state fishing license, 16
  tribal fishing permit, 16
fire safety
  burning trash, 9–10
  cooking, 10
  don't bring firewood from home, 10
fire watches See also forest fires
  Garnet Mountain fire lookout tower, 119
  McCart fire lookout (1940s) restoration, 150
  Porphyry Peak fire lookout tower, 65
first aid kit, 5–6
Fish Creek Campground, 27–29m
Fish Lake, 46
fishing permits See also specific campground
  state fishing license, 16
  tribal fishing permit, 16
Fishtrap Creek, 153
Flathead Indian Reservation, 16
Flathead Lake Monster legend, 15
Flathead Lake ("The Flathead"), 15–17m, 42
food
  fire safety, 9–10
  protecting from bears, 9
  tips on cooking, 9
forest fires See also fire watches
  August 1910 fire, 13
  Battle Creek recovery from 1988 fire, 165
  fire-ecology loop (Bass Creek Recreation Area)
    on, 137–138
  Moose Fire (2001), 18, 19
  Robert Fire (2003), 18
  Wedge Canyon fire (2003), 34
Forest Service Trail #308, 112
Fort Assinniboine, 77
Fort Belknap Indian Reservation, 80
Fort Owen State Park, 139
Fort Walla Walla, 158
fossils
  Lost Water Canyon, 92
  Makoshika State Park, 87
  petrified forest (Gallatin Petrified Forest
    Interpretive Trail #286), 125

Gallatin Canyon, 118, 121–123
Gallatin Petrified Forest Interpretive Trail #286,
  125
Gallatin River, 118, 119–120

Gallatin River Valley, 119
Garnet Mountain, 119
Garnet Mountain Trail, 119
George, James "Yankee Jim," 124
Giant Springs State Park, 61
Gibson Reservoir, 56, 57
Glacier Institute, 18, 20m
Glacier Lake Trail #3, 104
Glacier National Park
  Big Creek along the front of, 18
  controversy over oil drilling nearby, 33
  Going-to-the-Sun Road traversing, 45, 46, 47m
Glacier View Mountain Trail, 19
Going-to-the-Sun Road (Glacier National Park),
  45, 46, 47m
gold mining
  boom towns and ghost towns of, 134–135
  prospecting and, 80
  Welcome Creek (1888), 141
Golden Trout Lakes, 123
GPS entrance coordinates, 3
Graham Creek Trail #117, 101
Grasshopper Creek, 143
Grasshopper Creek boomtown (1862–65), 134
Gravelly Range, 131–132
Gravelly Range Road Backcountry, 131–132m
Graves, Fielding L., 135
Great Bear Wilderness area, 43
Great Falls Creek Trail #18, 101
Greenough, Ben, 103
Greenough family, 103
Greenough Lake Campground, 103–105m
Gros Ventre tribe, 80
Grouse Creek Trail #14, 101

Halfmoon Campground, 106–108m
Halfmoon Falls (or Big Timber Falls), 107
hammocks, 8
Hannan Gulch Trail #240, 56
Havre (Montana), 79
Hebgen Lake earthquake (1959), 127
Helena High School, 58
Helena National Forest, 58
Helena–Lewis and Clark National Forest, 67
Hi-Line region, 78, 79, 80
Hidden Lakes chain, 127
Highwoods Environmental Education Trail #452,
  71
Hill County Park, 77
History Rock Trail #424, 109
Holland Falls, 30, 31
Holland Lake Campground, 30–32m
Holland Lake Lodge, 30
Home Gulch Campground, 55–57m
Home Gulch–Lime Trail #267, 56

Homer Youngs Peak, 156
Hood Creek, 109, 111
Hood Creek Campground, 109–111*m*
Horner, Jack, 54
Hornet Peak Loop, 35
huckleberry-hunting country, 49
Huckleberry Mountain Trails, 29
Huckleberry Nature Trail, 29
Hungry Horse Dam, 42
Hungry Horse Reservoir, 42, 44*m*
Hyalite Lake, 110
Hyalite Peak, 109–110, 123

Ice Caves, 84, 85
insect repellent, 7

Jackson Hot Springs, 154
Joseph, Chief (1877), 77, 82, 158, 161
Jumbo Mountain, 162

Kading Cabin, 59
Kading Campground, 58–60*m*
Kings Hill Scenic Byway, 64
Kintla Lake Campground, 33–35*m*
Kishenehn Creek Trail, 34
KooKooSint Sheep Viewing Area, 49
Kootenai Creek Trail #53, 138
Kootenai National Forest, 21

Lake Alva Campground, 36–38*m*
Lake Como, 164, 166*m*
Lake Como National Recreational Loop Trail,
     164–165
Lake McDonald
     Fish Creek Campground, 27, 29*m*
     Sprague Creek Campground, 46–47*m*
Lake McDonald Lodge, 46
Lake Trail #184, 53–54
Lakota Sioux, 86
"Land of Bad Spirits" (Lakota Sioux), 86
Landusky, Pike, 80
Larabee Gulch, 59
laundry tips, 10
Lava Mountain Trail #244, 68
Leave No Trace practices, 10, 144
Lee Metcalf National Wildlife Refuge, 138
Lewis and Clark expedition, 81, 135, 147, 157, 158
Lewis and Clark Meeting Indians at Ross' Hole
     (Russell painting), 149
Lewis, Meriwether, 71
Limber Pine Campground, 104
Linderman, Bill, 103
Little Belt Mountains, 61, 64
Little Blackfoot River, 58–59
Little Blackfoot Valley, 58

Little Glacier Lake, 105
Little Lake Trail #87, 156
Little Rocky Mountains ("Fur Gaps"), 80
logging boom (early 1900s), 36–37
Logging Creek Campground, 61–63*m*
Logging Creek Road, 61
Lost Creek Falls, 146
Lost Creek State Park Campground, 146–148*m*
Lost Water Canyon, 91–92
Lower Lake Fork Trail #1, 105
Lower Miner Lakes, 155
"Lower Works" (1889) [copper ore processing],
     147

Madison Limestone Formation, 61
Madison River, 130–132*m*
Madison River Valley, 97
Makoshika State Park Campground,
     86–89*m*
Many Pines Campground, 64–66*m*
maps *See also specific campground*
     campground-layout, 3
     legend of, 3
marmots (vehicle damage caution), 105
Marshall, Bob, 73–74
Martin Creek, 149–151*m*
Martin Creek Campground, 149–151*m*
May Creek, 152–153
May Creek Cabin, 153
May Creek Campground, 152–154*m*
May Creek Trail #103, 153
McCart fire lookout (1940s) restoration, 150
McCart Lookout Trail, 150
Memorial Falls Trail #321, 65
Middle Fork Teton River Trail #108, 52
Miner Lake, 155–157*m*
Miner Lake Campground, 155–157*m*
Ming-Coulee Trail #307, 62
mining
     Bannack ghost town ("toughest town in the
          West"), 134–135
     Charter Oak Mine, 58
     Crystal Park and visitor crystal mining, 144
     gold prospecting, 80, 134–135, 141
     Grasshopper Creek boomtown (1862–1865)
          due to, 134
     "Lower Works" (1889) [processing copper ore],
          147
     New World Mining district, 115
     Smith Mine explosion (1943), 115
     Welcome Creek (1888), 141
Missouri River, 81
Mono Creek Campground, 144
Montana *See also specific state area*
     beauty and diversity of, 4

Montana *(Continued)*
  cell phone coverage in, 4
  Hi-Line region of, 78, 79, 80
  Lewis and Clark expedition through, 81, 135, 147, 157, 158
  logging boom (early 1900s) in, 36–37
  size and population of, 3
  weather extremes in, 4
Moose Creek, 149
Moose Creek Trail #168, 150
Moose Lake, 108
Morrell Falls National Recreation Trail #30, 38
Morrell Lake, 38
Mortimer Gulch Campground, 55–56
Mortimer Gulch Trail #252, 56
Mount Blackmore, 109
Mount Silcox Wildlife Management Area, 49
mountain lions, 6

National Register of Historic Places
  McCart fire lookout (1940s) restoration, 150
  Polebridge Mercantile, 34
National Wild and Scenic River System, 81
Native Americans
  Battle Ridge Pass skirmish between cowboys and, 94
  Blackfeet Indians, 55, 70
  Crow Indians, 90, 1060
  Custer's Little Big Horn (1876) defeat by, 77
  Flathead Indian Reservation, 16
  Fort Belknap Indian Reservation, 80
  Lakota Sioux on the "Land of Bad Spirits," 86
  Little Rocky Mountains named "Fur Gaps" by Gros Ventre tribe, 80
  Nez Perce Indians, 77, 82, 152, 156–157, 158, 161
  Rocky Boy's Reservation (Chippewa Cree tribe), 77, 78–79
  tribal fishing permit on reservations, 16
Natural Bridge, 100
Neil Creek Trail #654, 85
Neilhart (Montana), 64
Nelson, willie, 103
New World Mining district, 115
Nez Perce Indians
  Bear Paw Battlefield (Nez Perce National Historical Park), 77, 82
  Big Hole National Battlefield (Nez Perce War, 1877), 152, 156–157, 161
  Chief Joseph's surrender (1877), 77, 82, 158, 161
  Nez Perce Trail (1877) flight to Canada by, 156–157, 161
  Nez Perce War of 1877, 82, 152
North Central Montana
  Cave Mountain Campground, 52–54*m*
  Home Gulch Campground, 55–57*m*

Kading Campground, 58–60*m*
Logging Creek Campground, 61–63*m*
Many Pines Campground, 64–66*m*
Park Lake Campground, 67–69*m*
Thain Creek Campground, 70–72*m*
Wood Lake Campground, 73–75*m*
North Ford Deep Creek Trail #303, 62
North Ford Sun River Trail #201, 57
North Fork Highwood Creek Trail #423, 71
North Fork Teton Trail #107, 52–53
North Willow Creek Trail #301, 113
Northwest Montana
  Bad Medicine Campground, 12–14*m*
  Big Arm Unit–Flathead Lake State Park Campground, 15–17*m*
  Big Creek Campground, 18–20*m*
  Big Therriault Lake Campground, 21–23*m*
  Cut Bank Campground, 24–26*m*
  Fish Creek Campground, 27–29*m*
  Kintla Lake Campground, 33–35*m*
  Lake Alva Campground, 36–38*m*
  Pete Creek Campground, 39–41*m*
  Peters Creek Campground, 42–44*m*
  Sprague Creek Campground, 45–47*m*
  Thompson Falls State Park Campground, 48–50*m*
Northwest Peak Trail #169, 40
Northwest Peaks Scenic Area, 39–40

Old North Trail, 52
Old Snowdrift (white wolf), 70
Old Works Golf Course, 148
Owen, John, 138, 139

Paine Gulch Creek, 66
Paine Gulch Trail #737, 66
Palisade Falls National Recreation Trail, 111
Paradise Valley, 124
Park Lake, 67, 69*m*
Park Lake Campground, 67–69*m*
Pete Creek Campground, 39–41*m*
petrified forest (Gallatin Petrified Forest Interpretive Trail #286), 125
pets. *See specific campground*
Petty Ford Creek Trail #244, 74
Pine Butte Preserve, 53
Pioneer Mountains National Scenic Byway, 143
plant hazards, 7
Plenty Coups, Chief, 90
Plummer, Henry, 134, 135
poison ivy, 7
Polebridge Mercantile, 34
Porphyry Peak fire lookout, 65
Potosi Campground, 112–114*m*
Potosi Trail #303, 113
privacy rating, 1, 2

Pryor Mountain National Wild Horse Range, 91
Pryor Mountains, 90, 91

Quake Lake, 97, 98
quiet rating, 1, 2

Ralph Thayer Memorial National Recreation Trail, 19
rating system, 1–2
rattlesnakes, 6–7, 88
Red Lodge, 115–116
Red Lodge Valley, 103
rentals
    boats from Wade Lake Cabins, 128
    canoes (Seeley Lake), 37
    May Creek Cabin, 153
    yurt (Big Arm, Flathead Lake State Park), 16
reservation recommendations, 8
Reservoir Lake, 158–160m
Reservoir Lake Campground, 158–160m
Rock Creek, 105, 140–141, 165
Rock Creek and Forest Road 102, 140–142m
Rock Creek Canyon, 115
Rock Creek Trail #304, 113
Rock Island Lakes Trail #54, 156
Rocky Boy's Reservation (Chippewa Cree tribe), 77, 78–79
Rocky Mountain bighorn sheep
    Angle Draw herd, 149
    KooKooSint Sheep Viewing Area, 49
    Lost Creek State Park, 146
    Sun Canyon bighorn-sheep viewing area, 55
Rocky Mountain spotted fever, 7
Ross, Alexander, 158
Ross Creek Cedars Scenic Area, 12–13
Ross Creek Trail, 13
Ross' Hole (was Bitterroot Valley), 158
Ross Pass Connector Trail #551, 94
Ross Peak, 95
Russell, Charles M., 27, 71, 81, 149

Sacajawea Peak, 95
Sacajawea Peak Trail #509, 95
safety issues See also wildlife
    camp sites
        bear protection, 9, 81
        plant hazards, 7
        washing dishes/laundry/bathing, 10
    cell phone coverage, 4
    fires
        burning trash, 9–10
        cooking, 10
        don't bring firewood from home, 10
    first aid kit, 5–6
    weather, 4, 5, 8

Sage Creek Campground, 90–92m
St. Mary Peak Lookout #116, 138
St. Mary's Mission, 138
Sawtooth Lake Trail #195, 144
Sawtooth Mountain, 13
security rating, 1, 2
Seeley Lake, 37
Seeley Lake Ranger Station, 37
Seeley-Swan Valley, 30
Selway-Bitterroot Wilderness, 137, 165
Selway Mountain, 159
Servoss Mountain, 66
Sheridan Campground, 115–117m
Shonkin Sag (valley), 71
Shoreline Loop Trail #404, 84
Slag-a-melt Creek, 162
sleeping pads, 8
Sluice Boxes State Park, 61
Smith Creek Trail #215, 74
Smoky Rank National Recreation Trail, 19
Snake River country, 158
snakes, 6–7, 88
South Central Montana
    Battle Ridge Campground, 94–96m
    Beaver Creek Campground, 97–99m
    Falls Creek Campground, 100–102m
    Greenough Lake Campground, 103–105m
    Halfmoon Campground, 106–108m
    Hood Creek Campground, 109–111m
    Potosi Campground, 112–114m
    Sheridan Campground, 115–117m
    Spire Rock Campground, 118–120m
    Swan Creek Campground, 121–123m
    Tom Miner Campground, 124–126m
    Wade and Cliff Lakes Area Campgrounds, 127–129m
    West Fork Madison Dispersed Sites, 130–132m
South Willow Creek, 112
Southwest Montana
    Bannack State Park Campground, 134–136m
    Charles Waters Campground, 137–139m
    Dalles Campground, 140–142m
    Grasshopper Campground, 143–145m
    Lost Creek State Park Campground, 146–148m
    Martin Creek Campground, 149–151m
    May Creek Campground, 152–154m
    Miner Lake Campground, 155–157m
    Reservoir Lake Campground, 158–160m
    Three Frogs Campground, 164–166m
    Twin Lakes Campground, 161–163m
spaciousness rating, 1, 2
Spar Peak Trail, 13
Spire Rock Campground, 118–120m
Sportsman's Park, 153
Sprague Creek Campground, 45–47m

Spring Creek Trail #91, 142
Square Butte Natural Area ("Fort Mountain"), 71
state fishing license, 16
Storm Castle Creek, 118
Storm Castle Peak, 119
Storm Castle Trailhead, 119
Straight Creek Trail, 74
Sun River (Medicine River), 55, 57m
Sun River Wildlife Management Area, 55
Swan Creek, 121–123m
Swan Creek Campground, 121–123m
Swan Creek Trail #186, 123

Ten Lakes Scenic Area, 21
Tenderfoot Creek Trail System, 66
Tenderfoot Trail #342, 66
tent pitching tips, 8
Thain Creek Campground, 70–72m
Thain Creek (Espi-toh-tok), 70
Thain Creek Trail #411, 70–71
Thompson Falls, 49
Thompson Falls State Park Campground, 48–50m
Three Frogs Campground, 164–166m
ticks, 7
Tie Thru Trail #82, 22
Tobacco Root Range, 112–113
toilet facilities, 8–9
Tom Miner Basin, 125–126
Tom Miner Campground, 124–126m
tribal fishing permit, 16
Triple Divide Peak, 25
Twin Lakes, 161–163m
Twin Lakes Campground, 161–163m
Twin Lakes Trail #467, 162
Two Medicine Dinosaur Center (Bynum), 54

Upper Como Lake Campground, 164
Upper Kintla Lake, 34
Upper Miner Lake, 156
Upper Missouri River Breaks National Monument, 81
U.S. Forest Service (Darby Ranger Station Visitor Center and Museum), 165

Valley of the Moon Nature Trail, 141
Vinal–Mount Henry–Boulder National Recreation Trail #9, 39

Wade and Cliff Lakes Area Campgrounds, 127–129m
Wade Lake, 127–129m
waterfalls
   along Pete Creek, 39
   Big Timber Falls (or Halfmoon Falls), 107
   Double Falls, 74
   Holland Falls, 30, 31
   Lake Trail #184 (Cave Mountain Campground), 54m
   Lost Creek Falls, 146
   Morrell Falls, 38
   Thompson Falls, 49
watermelon snow (Chlamydomonas nivalis algae), 105
weather
   dressing for, 8
   seasonal extremes, 4, 5
Welcome Creek Wilderness Trailhead, 141
West Big Hole Mountains, 156
West Fork Madison Dispersed Sites, 130–132m
West Fork Madison River, 130–132m
West Fork Trail #144, 53
Whitetail (Forest Service site), 40
Wild and Scenic South Fork (Flathead River), 43
Wild Horse Island, 16–17
wildlife See also safety issues; specific campground
   hazards
      bears, 6, 9, 81
      marmots (causing vehicle damage), 105
      overview of different, 6
      rattlesnakes, 6–7, 88
      wolves, 6, 125–126
   Rocky Mountain bighorn sheep
      Angle Draw herd, 149
      KooKooSint Sheep Viewing Area, 49
      Lost Creek State Park, 146
      Sun Canyon bighorn-sheep viewing area, 55
wildlife areas See also specific campground area
   Charles M. Russell National Wildlife Refuge, 81
   Lee Metcalf National Wildlife Refuge, 138
   Mount Silcox Wildlife Management Area, 49
   Sun River Wildlife Management Area, 55
Willow Creek Anticline, 54
Windy Mountain Trail #454, 71
Wise River, 143
wolves
   be aware of the, 6
   controversy over reintroduced, 125–126
Wood Canyon, 73
Wood Lake, 73, 75m
Wood Lake Campground, 73–75m

Yaak Mercantile, 39
Yaak River, 39, 40
Yellowstone National Park, 115, 121, 124, 125
Yellowstone River, 124
Yellowstone Wildlife Sanctuary, 116
yurt rentals (Big Arm), 16

Zortman, Pete, 80